Obesity Management and Redux

Obesity Management and Redux™

Edited by

Stylianos Nicolaïdis

CNRS Directeur, College de France, Paris, France

ACADEMIC PRESS

San Diego London Boston New York
Sydney Tokyo Toronto

Copyright © 1997 by ACADEMIC PRESS

Academic Press, Inc.
525 B Street, Suite 1900, San Diego, California 92101-4495, USA
http://www.apnet.com

Academic Press Limited
24–28 Oval Road, London NW1 7DX, UK
http://www.hbuk.co.uk/ap/

ISBN 0-12-518170-1

Library of Congress Cataloging-in-Publication Data

Redux: a comprehensive overview / edited by Stylianos Nicolaidis.
    p.   cm.
    Includes index.
    ISBN 0-12-518170-1 (alk. paper). — ISBN 0-12-518170-1 (alk. paper)
    1. Dexfenfluramine—Congresses.   I. Nicolaidis, Stylianos.
    [DNLM: 1. Fenfluramine—pharmacology—congresses.
    2. Fenfluramine—therapeutic use—congresses.   3. Obesity—drug therapy—congresses.
QV 129 R321 1996]
RC628.R434   1996
616.3′98061—dc20
DNLM/DLC
for Library of Congress   96-36686
                                                                                      CIP

A catalogue record for this book is available from the British Library

Printed and bound by CPI Antony Rowe, Eastbourne

Contributors

M. Apfelbaum *Laboratoire de Nutrition, Hôpital Bichat, 16 rue Henri Huchard, 75018 Paris, France.*

R. L. Atkinson *Professor of Medicine and Nutritional Sciences, Chief of Clinical Nutrition, University of Wisconsin Medical School, Madison, WI 53706, USA.*

J. E. Blundell *BioPsychology Group, Department of Psychology, University of Leeds, Leeds LS2 9JT, UK.*

C. Bouchard *Laboratoire des Sciences de l'Activité Physique (LABSAP) Université Laval, Sainte Foy, Quebec G1K 7P4, Canada.*

G.A. Bray *Pennington Biomedical Research Center, Louisiana State University, 6400 Perkins Road, Baton Rouge, LA 70808-4124, USA.*

S. Caccia *Istituto di Ricerche Farmacologiche Mario Negri, Via Eritrea 62, 20157 Milan, Italy.*

B. Campbell *Servier Research and Development, Fulmer Hall, Windmill Road, Fulmer, Slough SL3 6HH, UK.*

B. Dard-Brunelle *Institut de Recherches Internationales Servier, 6 place des Pléiades, 92415 Courbevoie Cedex, France.*

M. Derôme-Tremblay *President, Servier Amérique, 22 rue Garnier, 92200 Neuilly sur Seine, France.*

R. Essner *President, Wyeth-Ayerst Laboratories, PO Box 8299, Philadelphia, PA 19101, USA.*

G. Faich *President, Outcomes Research Corporation, Bala Cynwyd, PA 19004, USA.*

S. Garattini *Istituto di Ricerche Farmacologiche Mario Negri, Via Eritrea 62, 20157 Milan, Italy.*

B. Guy-Grand *Department of Medicine and Nutrition, Hôtel-Dieu Hospital, Paris, France.*

M. Kalia *Professor of Neurosurgery, Jefferson Medical College, Thomas Jefferson University, Philadelphia, PA 19107, USA.*

N. Laudignon *Director, Metabolism Department, Institut de Recherches Internationales Servier, 6 Place des Pléiades, 92415 Courbevoie, France.*

S. A. Lorens *Professor of Pharmacology and Neuroscience, Department of Pharmacology and Experimental Therapeutics, Loyola University Chicago Medical Center, 2160 South First Avenue, Maywood, IL 60153, USA.*

T. Mennini *Istituto di Ricerche Farmacologiche Mario Negri, Via Eritrea 62, 20157 Milano, Italy.*

R. Y. Moore *Department of Psychiatry, Neurology and Neuroscience, Center for Neuroscience, University of Pittsburgh, Pittsburgh, PA 15261, USA.*

S. Nicolaïdis *CNRS Directeur, College de France, Paris, France.*

R. E. Noble *Director, Cathedral Hill Obesity Clinic, San Francisco, CA 94103, USA.*

J. P. O'Callaghan *Neurotoxicology Division, National Health and Environmental Effects Research Laboratory, US Environmental Protection Agency, Research Triangle Park, NC 27711, USA.*

M. Rebuffé-Scrive *Servier Amerique, 22 rue Garnier, 92200 Neuilly sur Seine, France.*

B. W. Sandage *Vice President, Research and Development, Interneuron Pharmaceuticals, Inc., One Ledgemont Center, 99 Hayden Avenue Suite 340, Lexington, MA 02173, USA.*

A. J. Stunkard *Professor of Psychiatry, Obesity Research Group, Department of Psychiatry, University of Pennsylvania, Philadelphia, PA 19104, USA.*

T. B. VanItallie *Professor Emeritus of Medicine, Columbia University, College of Physicians and Surgeons, New York, NY, USA.*

R. J. Wurtman *Cecil H. Green Distinguished Professor and Director, Clinical Research Center, Massachusetts Institute of Technology, Cambridge, MA 02139, USA.*

Preface

Obesity is a chronic disease that is increasing in prevalence. It contributes to worsening the overall morbidity and mortality in our societies and stigmatizes those with the condition. Obesity aggravates a number of co-morbid pathologies. Even a modest weight loss results in a significant improvement in both morbidity and mortality. To maintain the advantage of this weight loss prolonged treatment is often required. Unfortunately, facing this chronic disease the therapist is almost powerless. Very few options of treatment are available, particularly for sustained maintenance of weight loss and this is why appropriate pharmacotherapy is necessary. Today, the most efficient and tested long-term treatment of obesity calls on dexfenfluramine (Redux^{TM}), provided that certain conditions are taken into account.

This book has brought together internationally renowned specialists who, in 16 chapters, cover all aspects of obesity as a disease, its long-term treatment and the place of dexfenfluramine in this treatment. The spectrum of this book is particularly broad, providing an up-to-date survey of these topics covering a large array of information, from the most fundamental to the most applied.

To start with predisposition, a large number of individuals are susceptible to obesity. They are vulnerable to weight gain often due to a genetic trait and because the regulatory system is, in general, more permissive towards weight gain than weight loss. Indeed, phylogenetically, it was more appropriate for survival of the primitive *Homo sapiens* to set up mechanisms to protect against weight loss rather than weight gain, even though the latter could lead to obesity. After all, overweight in primitive conditions was often beneficial because it enabled survival during longer periods of food shortage. This trend, that still persists in the human genome, is exacerbated today because various environmental and nutritional factors tend to enhance intake, e.g. high palatability, high fat content, large and easily accessible meals flanked by snacks, low activity, anxiety and/or depression. These factors abound and converge to facilitate nonregulatory and excessive feeding and calorific drinking. Interestingly, it turns out that the main drug, dexfenfluramine, used in the treatment of obesity has been shown to counteract more or less all of these factors.

Dexfenfluramine acts mainly by reducing feeding because it speeds the onset of satiety, leading to a smaller size of meal. Dexfenfluramine predominantly reduces the consumption of both lipids and carbohydrates and of palatable snack craving. Dexfenfluramine enhances the onset of satiety also by slowing down gastric emptying together with the reduction of the overall rate of absorption of carbohydrate and fats.

However, appetite suppression is not the only mechanism by which a weight-reducing drug may bring about its leptogenic effect. It is well-established that bodyweight loss can be achieved by reducing nutrient intake and/or increasing energy expenditure. The best bodyweight controller would be the one that acts synergistically upon both intake, by decreasing it, and expenditure, by increasing it. Dexfenfluramine belongs to this class of compounds. Besides its anorexigenic action, it enhances metabolism. We have clearly established that dexfenfluramine mobilizes the fraction of lipids stored in adipocytes and, as a result, it provides an endogenous load of nutrients as if the subject had had a copious meal. This drug-induced excess of availability of metabolites of endogenous origin also enhances the metabolic rate in a similar way to the thermogenesis that is generated by a normal meal. In this respect dexfenfluramine classifies as a physiological regulator. This is why we used to refer to dexfenfluramine as a leptogenic (*leptos* = slim) rather than an anorexigenic drug.

Dexfenfluramines' central mechanism of action is well understood; it enhances serotoninergic (5-HT) transmission and function in the brain and probably elsewhere. This is true for fenfluramines' main action on feeding and bodyweight control but may extend to mood, immunity, sleep and memory or metabolism control as well. The action of dexfenfluramine and its central metabolite d-norphenfluramine is probably exerted via its impact on 5-HT 2c and also 5-HT 1b postsynaptic receptors. This direct action is reinforced by an indirect one that partially blocks the re-uptake of serotonin and thus enriches the synaptic cleft with this transmitter, a sort of feedback synergism. Dexfenfluramine acts on the 5-HT 1a presynaptic receptor as well. In addition, we have shown that dexfenfluramine enters in the cascade that uses cholecystokinine to promote satiety, another example of monoamine–peptide coaction that confers specificity to an otherwise ubiquitous neurotransmitter.

Dexfenfluramine is missing the sympathomimetic and dopaminergic properties that other molecules of this family exhibit. This accounts for the lack of addictive action of the drug.

This book also deals with the interesting and controversial question of effects of dexfenfluramine on brain chemistry that may produce adverse effects. Because the question of neurotoxicity has been raised, despite the 10-year use of the drug in more than 10 million patients, a comprehensive review of this occupies a large section of the book which carefully assesses all aspects of possible neurotoxicity of b-phenethylamines in general and of dexfenfluramine in particular. A considerable amount of work has been done during the last 30 years and dexfenfluramines' short term as well as long-term effects have been scrutinized using various procedures ranging from fine morphological and neurochemical techniques to behavioural and psychological tests.

From the overview presented in this book it appears that clinicians and researchers have devoted an exceptional number of investigations to dexfenfluramine in relation to obesity treatment and to its mechanism of action. This is as it should be, because even the most well-established mechanism of action of an active neurosubstance is being continuously challenged, completed or modified. Obviously, knowledge concerning widely used drugs has to be updated and added to continuously. Parallel or complementary mechanisms, new indications, short-term or long-term tolerance or risks have to be scrutinized. Therefore, the rule in pharmaceutical research should be to pursue investigating the properties of a drug as long as it is utilized in pharmacotherapy. This is precisely the philosophy concerning dexfenfluramine as is shown in the chapters of this book.

To conclude, as it is widely shown in the book, in spite of the small probability of adverse effects induced by this drug, pharmacotherapy should always be an adjunct to diet and other treatments including exercise and psychological support. This is why dexfenfluramine must only be used when the excess of bodyweight reaches abnormal percentages of body mass index, as the last chapters of this book clearly explain. It is also important that fenfluramine treatment must be discontinued in nonresponders. In effect, the main indication for dexfenfluramine (Redux^{TM}) treatment comes from the favourable benefit/risk ratio and from the despairing results of alternative therapies over the long-term struggle against obesity, this modern scourge of humanity.

Provided these precautions are respected dexfenfluramine-induced long-term bodyweight loss and maintenance will reduce other risk factors such as arteriosclerosis and cardiovascular morbidity and mortality.

Stylianos Nicolaïdis

Introduction

History of Dexfenfluramine

M. Derôme-Tremblay

President, Servier Amérique, 22 rue Garnier, 92200 Neuilly sur Seine, France

In over 30 years of therapeutic use, 60 million patients worldwide have been treated by dl fenfluramine and 10 million, so far, by dexfenfluramine. Dexfenfluramine, the 'product of the 80s', was the achievement of many years of research and development by the Servier Group and it continues to be the benchmark in the treatment of obesity and eating disorders.

The discovery in the 1960s of the first compound, the racemic dl fenfluramine came out of the search for an anorexigen compound lacking the effects of psycho-stimulants and sympathomimetic agents, such as amphetamines. At that time amphetamines were almost the only form of anorexigens available but the side effects (sympathomimetic activity, psycho-stimulant effects and addictive potential) made them difficult to use.

L. Beregi and Jacques Duhault, chemist and pharmacologist respectively, and their Servier research team, discovered the NCE, dl fenfluramine following a specific request by Dr Jacques Servier to look for such a compound. The structure was particularly interesting. Fenfluramine had an asymmetric carbon atom that presented a trifluoromethyl group substituted in the meta position of the core atom; a new pharmaco-chemical class. This compound was patented and marketed by Servier worldwide.

In 1965, Jacques Duhault carried out a study on the metabolism of dl fenfluramine in the rat. The study, backed by Michelle Boulanger, revealed the anti-obesity effects of the drug along with its anti-diabetic effects, an area in which Servier had always been active.

Studies on the isomers of fenfluramine began at the end of the 1960s and in the early 1970s, a new stage was broached with the demonstration of the effects

Obesity Management and Redux[T.M]
ISBN 0-12-518170-1

of dl and d on the serotoninergic system and its implication in the control of feeding behaviour. Numerous international scientists have further elucidated this mechanism of action. S. Garattini (Italy) and J. Blundell (England) are two pioneers in this field who have worked in close collaboration with our group in France and with Bruce Campbell and his team in the UK.

During the 1980s the field of neuroscience and metabolism exploded. As the study of feeding behaviour developed, it became difficult to isolate the study of food intake from the feeding behaviour that preceded or followed eating. Consequently *eating habits* encompassing behavioural and food intake parameters became a new study involving MIT researchers, Dick and Judith Wurtman. Meanwhile the group of S. Nicolaïdis (France) was revealing the metabolic and lipolytic properties of dexfenfluramine.

Research conducted on dexfenfluramine allowed Servier to specify the effect of dexfenfluramine on (1) general regulation of eating habits, (2) macronutrients selection, and (3) stress-induced eating.

Servier followed this research with numerous clinical trials involving international opinion leaders such as B. Guy-Grand (France) and N. Finer (UK) in Europe, G. Bray, T. VanItallie and R. Noble in the USA and J. P. Despres in Canada. Trials were carried out in Europe with Dr Nicole Laudignon and her team, in North America with myself and Dr Brigitte Riveling and in Australia for safety and efficacy purposes. Results demonstrated a progressive and regular weight loss with dexfenfluramine, which was maintained over the long term. The efficacy of dexfenfluramine was also proven in the most resistant cases of obesity with an improved adherence to a weight-loss programme. Also highlighted in these studies were the effects of dexfenfluramine with respect to risk factors associated with obesity, for example, diabetes, dyslipidaemia, hyperinsulinism, and X syndrome.

Dexfenfluramine is today the most studied molecule worldwide in the field of obesity.

On June 9th (1996), dexfenfluramine was the first anti-obesity drug treatment to be launched on the US market in 23 years. It was authorized by the Health Protection Branch of Canada last July 1996.

This was made possible due to the hundreds of people involved in all facets of this passionate development. More is to come!

Contents

Part I
Redux™: Pharmacological Profile

Part II
Methods for Assessing Neurochemical Changes and their Effect

Part III
Redux™: Therapeutic Efficacy

Part IV
Benefit/Risk Ratio of the Treatment of Obesity

New Trends in the Management of Obesity in the United States

George A. Bray

Pennington Biomedical Research Center, Baton Rouge, LA 70808-4124, USA

INTRODUCTION

For the first time in nearly a quarter century a new drug, dexfenfluramine (Redux[TM]), has been approved for the treatment of obesity. Equally important, the approval was for long-term use. As dexfenfluramine is being launched under the trade name Redux[TM], two other agents are moving toward FDA (US Food and Drug Administration) review and approval. The first is sibutramine, which will have the trade name Meridia[TM], and the second is orlistat, whose trade name is Xenical[TM].

These drugs are being developed and launched in a new environment for the treatment of obesity. The discovery of leptin as a product secreted by the fat cell that can reduce food intake and 'cure' the obese mouse of its obesity has made the study of obesity respectable (Zhang *et al.*, 1994; Campfield *et al.*, 1995; Halaas *et al.*, 1995; Pelleymounter *et al.*, 1995). It has also convinced the press and the public that obesity is not just a problem of willpower, but rather a metabolic problem that can be treated with medications. A second change in the environment for treatment of obesity is the already classic study of phentermine and fenfluramine, popularly called 'Fen-Phen', by Weintraub and his colleagues in 1992 (Weintraub *et al.*, 1992). This study, which lasted 4 years, demonstrated that long-term reduction in body weight was possible for many of the patients. Since this paper was published, the use of phentermine and fenfluramine has increased sharply. The number of prescriptions for fenfluramine increased by more than 400% between 1994 and 1995. The use of combination therapy for the treatment of obesity has a parallel in the treatment of hypertension. Two drugs are often better than one and side effects may be reduced by using combinations.

Obesity Management and Redux[TM]
ISBN 0-12-518170-1

Obesity is a chronic, stigmatized disease that is increasing in prevalence (Kuczmarski *et al.*, 1994). Like other chronic diseases, such as hypertension, effective treatment will mean chronic treatment. A corollary of this is that the public has to come to grips with the chronicity of the problem and that short-term treatment will not cure the problem. Another corollary of chronic disease treatment is that the risk of the treatment must be balanced against the risk of the disease.

Essentially all of the medications now approved by the FDA for treatment of obesity are β-phenethylamines and are chemically similar to amphetamine (Bray, 1993). Science and food writers thus frequently lump them together as 'amphetamine-like'. This is unfortunate, to say the least. It tars and feathers all drugs, even when they are not guilty. It is guilt by association. It is like calling all people 'men'. This is inaccurate and discredits and devalues women. The same is true for appetite-suppressant drugs when they are called 'amphetamine-like'. This 'negative' amphetamine halo conjures up concerns that are usually inappropriate.

Amphetamine, the first effective appetite suppressant, is a derivative of β-phenethylamine. Its name means *alpha-methyl (β)-phenethylamine* (Bray, 1995). It acts by releasing norepinephrine and dopamine. The appetite-suppressant effect is probably due to release of norepinephrine. The addictive properties, on the other hand, are due to the release of dopamine. The other sympathomimetic appetite-suppressant drugs such as phentermine and diethylpropion are also β-phenethylamines. However, they differ from amphetamine since they do not release dopamine. Thus, the potential for abuse of these drugs is very low.

DRUGS AROUND THE CORNER

Dexfenfluramine (Redux^{TM}), which has just been approved by the FDA, is also a β-phenethylamine. However, it is *not* a sympathomimetic. It does not release dopamine nor does it release norepinephrine. It works by releasing serotonin and partially blocking serotonin reuptake. In this sense it is much more like Prozac^{TM} or Zoloft^{TM} than amphetamine. We do not refer to Prozac or Zoloft as 'amphetamine-like' and it would be equally as irrational and inaccurate to refer to dexfenfluramine as 'amphetamine-like'. Indeed, a recent Advisory Committee to the FDA reviewed the potential for abuse of fenflur-amines. They could find no evidence for abuse in the past 20 years. On this basis they unanimously recommended that fenfluramine and its isomers be descheduled.

Dexfenfluramine (Redux^{TM}) has been extensively studied for more than a decade (Guy-Grand *et al.*, 1989). It produced a significantly greater weight loss than placebo in 18 of the 19 trials in which it has been used. More than twice as many patients treated with dexfenfluramine lose 10%, 15% or 20% of their body weight as compared with placebo-treated patients. The rate of initial weight loss is a good guide to whether patients will respond to dexfenfluramine. Patients losing less than 2 kg (4 lb) in 4 weeks have less than a 10% chance of losing 10% or more of their body weight at the end of 12 months of treatment. As a guideline these drugs, in my judgement, should be reserved for people who have a body mass index (BMI) of 30 kg m^{-2} or more or who have important health risks associated with their obesity.

The second drug which is just around the corner is sibutramine (Meridia^{TM}) (Ryan et al., 1995). It too is a β-phenethylamine, but is not amphetamine-like. There is no abuse potential for this drug. Clinical trials with sibutramine have been conducted in the USA and Europe. It produces a dose-related reduction in body weight. In a multicentre trial in the USA, weight loss is more than 5% greater than placebo with several doses of the drug. The drug works by blocking the reuptake of serotonin and norephrine. Thus, it is similar to the Phen-Fen combination of drugs.

The third drug in clinical trial is orlistat (Xenical^{TM}). This drug is not an appetite suppressant. Rather, it is a drug that inhibits pancreatic lipase. When fat is being digested, pancreatic lipase is the enzyme that breaks the dietary fat into the glycerol and fatty acids. If this lipase is completely blocked fat will not be digested. The faecal loss of fat is related to both the amount of drug and the amount of fat in the diet. On a very low fat diet the drug has little effect. In clinical trials in Europe, the drug has produced more weight loss than placebo. Its major side effects are related to incomplete digestion of fat (Drent et al., 1995).

The fourth drug in this group is ephedrine. On its own, ephedrine is not significantly different from placebo in long- or short-term trials. However, one double-blind placebo-controlled trial from Europe has shown that ephedrine in combination with caffeine is significantly more effective in producing weight loss over an entire year (Astrup et al., 1992).

DRUGS ON THE HORIZON

As the drugs described above enter the marketplace, several others are right behind. Based on a review of this problem for the *Annals of Internal Medicine* (Bray, 1993), I have grouped these drugs into three categories based on their mechanism of action (Table 1). The first group includes those drugs which reduce food intake; the second group includes drugs which affect gastric emptying or the way in which nutrients are metabolized; and the final group is the drugs which stimulate thermogenesis.

Table 1
New drugs for obesity

Mechanism of action	Drugs
Reduce food intake or shift nutrient preferences	Serotonin-like drugs
	Opioid antagonists
	α-2 antagonists
	α-1 agonists
	Cholecystokinin
	NPY antagonists
	Enterostatin
	Galanin antagonists
	Leptin
	GLP-1
Inhibit gastric emptying or shift nutrient partitioning	Chlorocitrate
	Acarbose
	Orlistat
	Olestra
	β-adrenergic agonists
	Androgens/oestrogens
	Glucocorticoids
Stimulate thermogenesis	β-3 agonists
	Thyroid analogues
	Uncoupling agents

*Adapted from Bray, 1993

Increasing interest in drug treatment for obesity is spurred by the greater acceptance that obesity, like hypertension, is a disease. This attitude, however, is out of phase with many of the regulatory agencies in states across the USA. Florida, for example, held a symposium before its members on obesity. Several experts were asked to testify. Massachusetts, one of the most restrictive states, has allowed use of these drugs for the first time in more than a decade. Other states are also evaluating their guidelines. In this rapidly changing environment it is likely to be the obese patient who will be the eventual winner.

REFERENCES

Astrup A, Breum L, Toubro S, Hein P, Quaade F (1992) The effect and safety of an ephedrine/caffeine compound compared to ephedrine, caffeine and placebo in obese subjects on an energy restricted diet. A double blind trial. *Int J Obesity* 16: 269–277.

Bray GA (1993) Use and abuse of appetite-suppressant drugs in the treatment of obesity. *Ann Intern Med* **119**: 707–713.

Bray GA (1995) Evaluation of drugs for treating obesity. *Obesity Res* **3**: 425S–434S.

Campfield LA, Smith FJ, Guisez Y, Devos R, Burn P (1995) Recombinant mouse OB protein: Evidence for a peripheral signal linking adiposity and central neural networks. *Science* **269**: 546–549.

Drent ML, Larsson I, Williamson T *et al.* (1995) Orlistat (RO-18-0647), a lipase inhibitor, in the treatment of human obesity: A multiple dose study. *Int J Obesity* **19**: 221–226.

Guy-Grand B, Apfelbaum M, Crepaldi G, Gries A, Lefebvre P, Turner P (1989) International trial of long-term dexfenfluramine in obesity. *Lancet* **ii**: 1142–1144.

Halaas JL, Gajiwala KS, Maffei M *et al.* (1995) Weight-reducing effects of the plasma-protein encoded by the obese gene. *Science* **269**: 543–546.

Kuczmarski RJ, Flegal KM, Campbell SM, Johnson CL (1994) Increasing prevalence of overweight among US adults: The National Health and Nutrition Examination Surveys, 1960 to 1991. *J Am Med Assoc* **272**: 205–211.

Pelleymounter MA, Cullen MJ, Baker MB *et al.* (1995) Effects of the obese gene-product on body-weight regulation in OB/OB mice. *Science* **269**: 540–543.

Ryan DH, Kaiser P, Bray GA (1995) Sibutramine: A novel new agent for obesity treatment. *Obesity Res* **4**: 553S–559S.

Weintraub M, Sundaresan PR, Schuster B *et al.* (1992) Long term weight control: the National Heart, Lung and Blood Institute funded multimodal intervention study. I–VII. *Clin Pharmacol Ther* **51**: 581–646.

Zhang YY, Proenca R, Maffei M, Barone M, Leopold L, Friedman JM (1994) Positional cloning of the mouse obese gene and its human homolog. *Nature* **372**: 425–432.

The Impact of Obesity and the Introduction of Redux™ in the United States

Robert Essner

President, Wyeth-Ayerst Laboratories, Philadelphia, PA 19101-1245, USA

In 1990, the total cost of obesity in the United States reached almost $70 billion. Approximately $46 billion was spent to treat obesity-related diseases such as cardiovascular disease, diabetes, musculoskeletal disease, gallbladder disease, and some cancers. Another $23 billion was spent on indirect costs such as days lost from work or costs arising from death caused by obesity-related diseases (Wolf and Colditz, 1994). Obesity is a contributing risk factor for four of the seven leading causes of death in the United States (Colditz *et al.*, 1995; Gordon and Kannel, 1976; Hubert *et al.*, 1983; Lew and Garfinkel, 1979; U.S. Bureau of the Census, 1995).

There is an evolution of understanding about managing obesity in the United States. People are much better informed about healthcare in general and obesity in particular. We now know that obesity is rooted in our genetic makeup, environment, culture, socioeconomic and psychological backgrounds.

Our culture, as demonstrated by the spotlight most consumer publications put on obesity, is fascinated by the idea of losing weight. Obesity is a battle that if we are not personally fighting ourselves, we certainly know someone who is. In any given year, 40% of all women in the United States and 25% of all men are on a weight-loss regime. Unfortunately, within a few years, 90% of these dieters regain all the weight that was lost (Brody, 1992; National Institutes of Health, 1992).

Even with this intense interest in the health consequences of obesity, physicians very often failed to manage obesity in clinical practice, because they simply had no suitable tools to help them with the recidivism.

Redux™ is the first new weight-loss agent in over twenty years, and the

Obesity Management and Redux™
ISBN 0-12-518170-1

only one indicated for maintenance of weight loss. The introduction of Redux™ represents more than simply the availability of a new drug. It also represents a change in attitude toward obesity and its management. In this respect Redux™ definitely contributes to the understanding of obesity as a chronic medical condition that may require pharmacological intervention.

Although weight management is in some sense unique, there are important lessons to be learned from products in other therapeutic categories. Hypertension, for example, has a history very similar to weight management. At one time, there were few therapeutic options for patients. Hypertension and the associated risks were seriously undertreated or treated by unsatisfactory measures. The advent of antihypertensive agents created a market that included routine patient screening and counselling. Over the last two decades, the number of patients diagnosed and treated has at the very least doubled.

Another similar therapeutic category is hyperlipidaemia. The new therapeutic modalities, the HMG Co-A reductase synthesis inhibitors, have been found not only to reduce cholesterol, but also to prevent heart attack and prolong life. As a result, the number of diagnosed and treated instances have increased rapidly over the last few years.

Drugs like Redux™ are the catalysts that can help improve the management of obesity by providing a tool for physicians to manage the condition in a responsible manner. Redux™ promotion to healthcare professionals in the United States specifically addresses the following points:

- Appropriate candidates for Redux™ therapy are clearly identified. Redux™ is indicated for the obese patients who are 30% over their ideal weight or patients with additional risk factors who are approximately 20% over ideal weight. Redux™ is not for cosmetic weight loss.
- The link between obesity and various comorbid conditions presents a strong rationale for the use of Redux™. A modest weight loss of 5% to 10% can improve blood pressure, blood sugar, and cholesterol levels in obese patients with hypertension, diabetes or hyperlipidaemia.
- The risks associated with Redux™ therapy are proactively communicated.
- The efficacy profile of Redux™ is presented, accurately, fostering realistic expectations of the drug's performance.
- Redux™ is distanced from the negative image surrounding amphetamines. This is accomplished in two ways: by emphasizing its mechanism of action through serotonin but not DA release and re-uptake inhibition, and by highlighting the fact that Redux™ is not associated with addictive behaviour.
- Support programmes are provided, which include patient literature and collaborative efforts with successful consumer programs such as Weight Watchers. Materials from the American Diabetes Association, Shape-Up America, and the American Heart Association are provided among others.

In conclusion, from the set of data in the literature, priority is being given to promote Redux™ responsibly, ensuring long-term success of obesity management.

REFERENCES

Brody JE (1992) Panel criticizes weight-loss programs. *New York Times*, April 2.

Colditz GA, Willet WC, Rotnitzky A and Manson JE (1995) Weight gain as a risk factor for clinical diabetes mellitus in women. *Ann. Intern. Med.* **122**: 481–488.

Gordon T and Kannel WB (1976) Obesity and cardiovascular disease: the Framingham Study. *Clinics in Endocrinology and Metabolism.* **5**(2): 367–375.

Hubert HB, Feinleib M, McNamara PM and Castelli WP (1983) Obesity as an independent risk factor for cardiovascular disease: A 26-year follow-up of participants in the Framingham Heart Study. *Circulation* **67**(5) 968–976.

Lew EA and Garfinkel L (1979) Variations in mortality by weight among 750,000 men and women. *J. Chron. Dis.* **32**: 563–576.

National Institutes of Health (1992) *Technology Assessment Statement on Methods for Voluntary Weight Loss and Control.*

U.S. Bureau of the Census (1995) *Statistical Abstract of the United States,* 115th edn.

Wolf AM and Colditz GA (1994) The cost of obesity—the US perspective. *Pharma-Economics* **5**(Suppl. 1): 34–37.

Part I

Redux™: Pharmacological Profile

The Pharmacology of Dexfenfluramine

Richard J. Wurtman

Cecil H. Green Distinguished Professor and Director, Clinical Research Center, Massachusetts Institute of Technology, Cambridge, MA 02139, USA

INTRODUCTION

The dexfenfluramine molecule resembles *d*-amphetamine in that it contains a substituted phenylethylamine moiety (Fig. 1). Indeed this similarity – and the assumption that such molecules would have amphetamine-like effects on

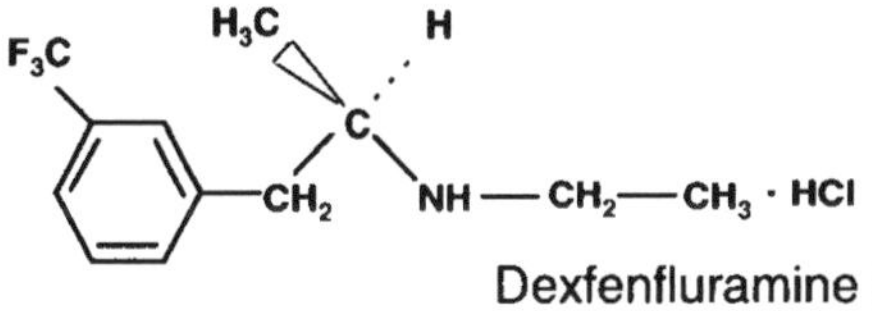

Dexfenfluramine (DF)

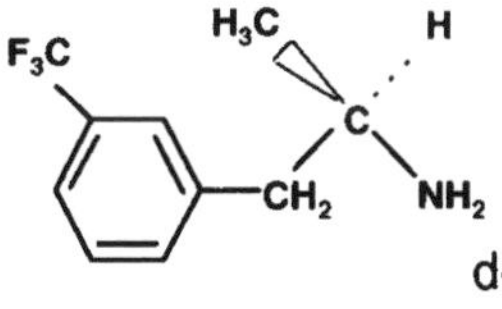

d-Norfenfluramine (dNF)

Fig. 1. Chemical structures of dexfenfluramine and *d*-norfenfluramine. Dexfenfluramine is a substituted phenethylamine also containing a trifluorocarbon moiety – which probably imparts specificity for serotonin-binding macromolecules – and an ethylamine chain. The ethyl portion is removed when dexfenfluramine is metabolized, yielding *d*-*nor*fenfluramine. Unchanged dexfenfluramine blocks the reuptake of serotonin from the synapse; *d*-norfenfluramine acts both to release serotonin into synapses and to activate directly certain postsynaptic serotonin receptors. The fenfluramine molecules contain an asymmetric carbon atom, indicated on the diagram by the triangle and dotted line; hence there can be both a dexfenfluramine and an *l*-fenfluramine.

Obesity Management and Redux^{T.M}
ISBN 0-12-518170-1

weight loss – were what led to fenfluramine's synthesis in the first place. However this chemical resemblance is *all* that dexfenfluramine shares with *d*-amphetamine: dexfenfluramine is not an amphetamine-like drug. Rather, it is a *serotoninergic* agent, which acts in three ways, described below, to enhance serotonin-mediated neurotransmission in the brain. *d*-Amphetamine, in contrast, is a *dopaminergic* drug, and as such it primarily affects appetite, not satiety, and decreases the consumption of all macronutrients and not principally carbohydrates (and fats). Because *d*-amphetamine acts via dopamine, its use is associated with habituation and tolerance, as well as, in some patients, psychiatric symptoms. Although fenfluramines were initially described as 'sympathomimetic amines' – and fenfluramine itself mistakenly continues to be listed as such in the *Physician's Desk Reference* – dexfenfluramine has no sympathomimetic properties; its administration tends to *lower* blood pressure, not raise it.

Fenfluramine contains an asymmetric carbon atom (Fig. 1), thus both a *d*-isomer (dexfenfluramine) and an *l*-isomer exist. The *d*-isomer has all of the therapeutic activity, while the *l*-isomer, which blocks dopamine-mediated neurotransmission, can produce tiredness, similar to that seen after other dopamine antagonists. This tiredness can usually be ameliorated by concurrently administering an additional drug, for example phentermine, which activates brain dopamine release and/or dopamine receptors. With dexfenfluramine, the addition of an amphetamine-like dopaminergic drug is unnecessary.

The principal metabolite of dexfenfluramine, comprising perhaps 33% of the total fenfluramine in brains of people taking the drug, is dex*nor*fenfluramine (Garattini and Mennini, this volume) (Fig. 1). This compound has important pharmacological properties, mediating two of the three processes through which dexfenfluramine enhances serotonin-mediated neurotransmission. It releases serotonin from presynaptic terminals directly into synapses, and it also activates the postsynaptic 5-HT-2C receptors (Garattini and Mennini, this volume) which probably underlie the drug's weight-reducing effects (Spedding *et al.*, 1996). Dexfenfluramine itself acts as a serotonin-reuptake blocker. It seems extraordinarily fortunate that all three of the neurochemical actions of dexfenfluramine and its main central nervous system (CNS) metabolite, dexnorfenfluramine, have the same net neurochemical effect: promotion of serotonin-mediated neurotransmission.

The weight loss associated with dexfenfluramine treatment (Guy-Grand *et al.*, 1989) principally reflects decreased food intake (Wurtman and Wurtman, 1989) (Fig. 2); the drug also probably causes a small (100 calorie day^{-1}) increase in calorie utilization. Dexfenfluramine – and serotonin, through which it acts – decreases food consumption in two ways. First, it speeds the onset of satiety (Blundell, this volume), such that patients elect to

Effects of Serotonin and Dexfenfluramine on Food Intake and Energy Utilization

- ◆ ⬆ Serotonin
    - – Increases satiety
    - – Suppresses food craving
    - – Increases basal energy utilization
- ◆ Dexfenfluramine
    - – Reduces daily caloric intake 400-600 kcal/day
    - – Increases basal energy expenditure 100 kcal/day

Fig. 2.   Mechanisms of action of serotonin and dexfenfluramine in affecting body weight.

eat smaller portions of food than would otherwise be the case. Second, it selectively suppresses the desire of many patients to overeat carbohydrates – particularly carbohydrate-rich snack foods which usually are also rich in fats (Wurtman and Wurtman, 1989). The 'carbohydrate craving' apparently results from the patient's having learned that high-carbohydrate, low-protein foods can improve his or her mood, probably by increasing synaptic levels of serotonin. (The carbohydrates elicit the secretion of insulin, which increases the 'plasma tryptophan ratio' – the ratio of the plasma tryptophan concentration to the summed concentrations of other large neutral amino acids which compete with tryptophan for uptake into the brain. The resulting rise in brain tryptophan levels enhances the substrate saturation of the enzyme tryptophan hydroxylase, increasing the production and release of serotonin.) Dexfenfluramine reduces body weight in obese patients whether or not they are also 'carbohydrate cravers'; however, it may be somewhat more effective in the 'cravers'. Its use reduces daily calorie intake in patients who are 20–30% overweight by about 500–600, half from meals and half from snacks. The net decrease in available calories (600–700 day^{-1}) is compatible with a weekly weight loss of 1–2 lb (0.05–1 kg). It should be noted that a number of diseases and conditions – like seasonal depression, smoking withdrawal, the premenstrual syndrome and stress – also seem to cause 'carbohydrate craving', which predisposes to obesity. A serotoninergic drug like dexfenfluramine can protect the patient against weight *gain* by its carbohydrate-like effect on serotonin-mediated neurotransmission. Dexfenfluramine, unlike the amphetamines, apparently does not significantly reduce dietary protein intake (Wurtman and Wurtman, 1979), a desirable property for a drug that can be administered long-term.

REFERENCES

Guy-Grand B, Crepaldi G, Lefebvre P, Apfelbaum M, Gries A, Turner P (1989) International trial of long-term dexfenfluramine in obesity. *Lancet* **ii**: 1142–1144.

Spedding M, Ouvry C, Millan M, Duhault J, Dacquet C, Wurtman RJ (1996) Neural control of dieting. *Nature* **380**: 488.

Wurtman JJ, Wurtman RJ (1979) Fenfluramine and other serotoninergic drugs depress food intake and carbohydrate consumption while sparing protein consumption. *Curr Med Res Opin* **6**: 28–33.

Wurtman RJ, Wurtman JJ (1989) Carbohydrates and depression. *Sci Am* January: 68–75.

Neurochemical Mode of Action of Drugs which Modify Feeding through the 5-HT System

S. Garattini and T. Mennini

Istituto di Ricerche Farmacologiche Mario Negri, Via Eritrea 62, 20157 Milan, Italy

Increasing evidence from animal studies indicates serotonin (5-hydroxy-tryptamine, 5-HT) as a key mediator in the control of food intake (Samanin, 1983; Leibowitz, 1990). Serotonin reduces food intake, especially of carbo-hydrates (Leibowitz, 1990), and reduced availability of 5-HT at postsynaptic receptors in relevant brain areas increases food intake in satiated rats by stimulation of presynaptic 5-HT_{1A} receptors (Dourish *et al.*, 1985; Bendotti and Samanin, 1987).

Many drugs that increase serotonergic neurotransmission in the brain exert anorectic activity at doses that do not stimulate animal behaviour, in a different way from those acting on catecholamines (Bizzi *et al.*, 1970; Garattini *et al.*, 1978). These drugs accumulate in the brain, and give rise to metabolites (see Fig. 1) that often retain the anorectic effect of the parent compound (Garattini *et al.*, 1989, 1991). This short review focuses on the activity on food intake shown by agents that affect 5-HT transmission.

There is no evidence that blocking the metabolism of 5-HT by monoamine oxidase inhibitors reduces food intake. Inhibition of 5-HT uptake is another way of increasing extracellular 5-HT concentrations. Agents like fluoxetine, sertraline, paroxetine and fluvoxamine all induce hypophagia in rodents (Caccia *et al.*, 1993), presumably by inhibiting 5-HT uptake by nerve terminals. A single anorectic dose of these drugs lowers 5-HIAA concen-trations in the cortex, hippocampus and striatum; only fluvoxamine and sertraline raised 5-HT in the cortex by about 20% (Garattini *et al.*, 1992; Caccia *et al.*, 1993). However, a dissociation between 5-HT uptake inhibition

Obesity Management and Redux[TM]
ISBN 0-12-518170-1

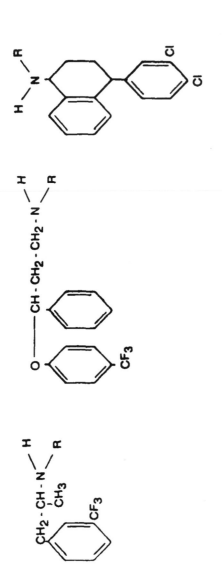

Fig. 1.   Chemical structures of dexfenfluramine (d-fenfluramine), fluoxetine, sertraline and their respective metabolites.

and anorexia has been suggested since the brain concentrations of all these drugs and their active metabolites are several hundred times the IC_{50} for inhibiting 5-HT uptake *in vitro* (Samanin and Garattini, 1990; Garattini *et al.*, 1992). These discrepancies may be explained by recent results with citalopram, showing that its hypophagic effect in rats, which was blocked by the non-selective 5-HT antagonist metergoline, was reduced by the selective 5-HT_{1A} receptor agonist 8-OH-DPAT (Grignaschi *et al.*, 1996). In contrast, the selective 5-HT_{1A} antagonist WAY-100635, injected into the nucleus raphe dorsalis, potentiated the effect of citalopram on food intake and on the extracellular dialysate 5-HT (Grignaschi *et al.*, 1996). Thus, citalopram reduces food intake by acting on 5-HT neurons originating from the dorsal raphe, and its effect can be modulated by changes in the activity of presynaptic 5-HT_{1A} receptors. The usefulness of combinating selective 5-HT uptake inhibitors with a 5-HT_{1A} antagonist in the treatment of clinical obesity remains to be explored.

The involvement of the 5-HT system in the activity of fluoxetine and sertraline is not clear, since there are conflicting results about the effect of 5-HT receptor antagonists or neurotoxins in antagonizing their hypophagic effects (Samanin and Garattini, 1993). *In vitro* findings on brain synaptosomes suggest that fluoxetine (Gobbi *et al.*, 1995), sertraline and paroxetine – but not citalopram or indalpine – displace ^{3}H-5HT from synaptic vesicles into the cytoplasm (Garattini, 1995), where it is deaminated with the subsequent efflux of ^{3}H-5-HIAA. Consistently, when fluoxetine is injected twice daily for 21 days in rats at doses of 7.5 or 15 mg kg^{-1} i.p. there is a dose-dependent decrease of 5-HT in the cortex, hippocampus and striatum at short (1 h) or long (1 week) times after the last injection (Caccia *et al.*, 1993).

Increasing 5-HT release is another mechanism by which anorectic agents can raise extracellular 5-HT. The most widely studied compounds acting on this mechanism are dexfenfluramine (dF) and its metabolite, dexnorfenfluramine (dNF). This metabolite contributes to, but does not explain, the anorectic effect of dF in rats and other animal species, with the exception of guinea pigs, where dF seems to be a pro-drug of dNF (Mennini *et al.*, 1991). Both compounds *in vitro* inhibit 5-HT reuptake and stimulate its release from brain synaptosomes of different animal species (Mennini *et al.*, 1991, 1996a), at concentrations compatible with their brain levels after anorectic doses, suggesting that these effects may have significance *in vivo*.

The nor-metabolite is less effective than dF on 5-HT uptake but shows the same activity in enhancing 5-HT release. Important differences between dF and dNF are that the metabolite releases 5-HT also from synaptosomes of reserpinized rats (Mennini *et al.*, 1981), i.e. from a non-vesicular pool; and that it enhances ^{3}H-dopamine release from striatal synaptosomes (Mennini *et al.*, 1996b). In addition dNF has affinities varying from 120 to 590 nM for 5-HT_{2C} receptors in different animal species (Mennini *et al.*, 1991), suggesting it might also act as a direct 5-HT_{2C} agonist (Gibson *et al.*, 1993) in rodents (Mennini *et al.*, 1991) and primates (Mennini *et al.*, 1996a).

The effect of dF (and dNF) on 5-HT uptake *in vitro* is probably due to competition of the drug with the same 5-HT transporter. In fact $^3\text{H-dF}$ itself is actively taken up by synaptosomes (Garattini *et al.*, 1989). This uptake is blocked by 5-HT and 5-HT uptake inhibitors like fluoxetine (Garattini *et al.*, 1989). On the other hand, 5-HT uptake inhibitors block the release of synaptosomal 5-HT *in vitro* (Maura *et al.*, 1982; Gobbi *et al.*, 1992) and the depletion of brain indoles *in vivo* (Ghezzi *et al.*, 1973; Sabol *et al.*, 1992) induced by dF. The 5-HT releasing activity of low doses of dF *in vitro* is exocytotic-like, in that it is dependent on extracellular Ca^{2+} (Gobbi *et al.*, 1992, 1993a), blocked by tetanus toxin (Gobbi *et al.*, 1993b) and by antagonists of the P-type, and to a less extent the N-type, calcium channels (Frittoli *et al.*, 1994). Differently from K^+-induced $^3\text{H-5-HT}$ release, the Ca^{2+}-dependent dF-induced $^3\text{H-5-HT}$ release can be blocked by inhibitors of serotonin uptake (Gobbi *et al.*, 1992), and by methiotepine, flunarizine and trifluperazine, which also block the *in vivo* dF-induced lowering of 5-HT concentrations (Mennini *et al.*, 1996b).

These results suggest that, at low concentrations, dF enters the nerve ending through the 5-HT uptake carrier, and that it activates an intracellular target, sensitive to methiotepine, trifluperazine and flunarizine, that induces the influx of Ca^{2+} through the P-type calcium channels. At a higher concentration, the release is less Ca^{2+}-dependent and consists mainly of metabolized 5-HT (Gobbi *et al.*, 1992), suggesting that dF enters by passive diffusion and displaces 5-HT from vesicles, for which both dF and dNF have low affinity (Garattini *et al.*, 1978, 1992). In line with these *in vitro* mechanisms, *in vivo* dF raises the extracellular concentration of 5-HT measured by brain microdialysis (Schwartz *et al.*, 1989) and the extracellular concentration of 5-HIAA measured by pulse voltametry (De Simoni *et al.*, 1988).

Dexfenfluramine therefore increases serotonergic transmission both indirectly, by inhibiting 5-HT uptake and enhancing its release, and directly, by its metabolite's action on 5-HT_{2C} receptors. This makes it difficult to assess the contribution of presynaptic mechanisms in dF-induced hypophagia, which depend on the animal species and the route of administration. For instance, after i.p. injection of anorectic doses of dF in rats, the parent drug and metabolite are present in the brain to almost the same extent (Mennini *et al.*, 1991). Therefore, attempts to impair the presynaptic components of dF-induced hypophagia (Oluyomi *et al.*, 1994; Raiteri *et al.*, 1995) do not reduce the anorectic effect of dF, since activation of 5-HT_{2C} receptors by dNF could prevail. This mechanism becomes even more important after oral administration of dF (McCann *et al.*, 1995), when the brain concentration of metabolite greatly exceeds that of the parent compound (Caccia *et al.*, 1992). In addition the presence of 5-HT fibres resistant to *p*-chlorophenylalanine

(Tohyama *et al.*, 1988) may explain why dF-induced hypophagic effects are not antagonized in rats treated with the inhibitor of 5-HT synthesis (Oluyomi *et al.*, 1994).

As to the role of 5-HT receptor subtypes in the control of food intake, some information has been obtained with dF. The feeding patterns of rats treated with dF (Grignaschi and Samanin, 1992) show that metergoline can antagonize all the parameters affected by dF (total food intake, meal size and eating rate). ($\pm$)Cyanopindolol, an antagonist of 5-HT_{1A} and 5-HT_{1B} receptors, reduced the effects of dF on total intake and meal size but not eating rate. Ritanserin, an inhibitor of 5-HT_2 receptors, reduced only the effect on the rate of eating. The involvement of 5-HT_{1A-B} and 5-HT_{2C} receptors in the control of food intake has been further established by the use of selective agonists, and by a recent report of overweight and eating disorders in mice lacking the 5-HT_{2C} receptors (Tecott *et al.*, 1995).

In conclusion, it appears that activation of 5-HT_{1B} and 5-HT_{2C} receptors – either directly, or by inhibiting 5-HT reuptake and/or enhancing its release – are the most important mechanisms through which drugs influence food intake by acting on the serotonergic system.

REFERENCES

Bendotti C, Samanin R (1987) *Life Sci* **41**: 635.
Bizzi A *et al.* (1970) In: Costa E and Garattini S (eds) *Amphetamines and Related Compounds*. New York, Raven Press: 570.
Caccia S *et al.* (1992) *Xenobiotica* **22**: 217.
Caccia S *et al.* (1993) *Br J Pharmacol* **110**: 355.
De Simoni MG *et al.* (1988) *Eur J Pharmacol* **153**: 295.
Dourish CT *et al.* (1985) *Psychopharmacology* **86**: 197.
Frittoli E *et al.* (1994) *Neuropharmacology* **33**: 833.
Garattini S (1995) *Obesity Res* **3** (suppl. 4): 463S.
Garattini S *et al.* (1978) In: Garattini S and Samanin R (eds) *Central Mechanisms of Anorectic Drugs*. New York, Raven Press: 127.
Garattini S *et al.* (1989) *Br J Psychiat* **155** (suppl. 8): 41.
Garattini S *et al.* (1991) In: Rothwell NJ and Stock MJ (eds) *Obesity and Cachexia: Physiological Mechanisms and New Approaches to Pharmacological Control*. Chichester, Wiley: 227.
Garattini S *et al.* (1992) *Int J Obes* **16** (suppl. 3): S43.
Ghezzi D *et al.* (1973) *Eur J Pharmacol* **24**: 205.
Gibson EL *et al.* (1993) *Eur J Pharmacol* **242**: 83.
Gobbi M *et al.* (1992) *Naunyn Schmiedeberg's Arch Pharmacol* **345**: 1.
Gobbi M *et al.* (1993a) *Eur J Pharmacol* **238**: 9.
Gobbi M *et al.* (1993b) *Neurosci Lett* **151**: 205.
Gobbi M *et al.* (1995) *Life Sci* **56**: 785.
Grignaschi G and Samanin R (1992) *Eur J Pharmacol* **212**: 287.
Grignaschi G *et al.* (1996) *Br J Pharmacol* (submitted).
Leibowitz SF (1990) *Drugs* **39** (suppl. 3): 33.

Maura G et al. (1982) Neurochem Int 4: 219.

McCann UD et al. (1995) Eur J Pharmacol 283: R5.

Mennini T et al. (1981) Neurochem Int 3: 289.

Mennini T et al. (1991) Naunyn Schmiedeberg's Arch Pharmacol 343: 483.

Mennini T et al. (1996a) Naunyn Schmiedeberg's Arch Pharmacol 353: 641.

Mennini T et al. (1996b) Pharmacol Biochem Behav 53: 155.

Oluyomi AO et al. (1994) Eur J Pharmacol 264: 111.

Raiteri M et al. (1995) J Pharm Exp Ther 273: 643.

Sabol KE et al. (1992) Brain Res 585: 421.

Samanin R (1983) In: Curtis-Prior PB (ed.) Biochemical Pharmacology of Obesity. Amsterdam, Elsevier: 339.

Samanin R and Garattini S (1990) In: Wurtman RJ and Wurtman JJ (eds) Nutrition and the Brain. New York, Raven Press: 8: 163.

Samanin R and Garattini S (1993) Pharmacol Toxicol 73: 63.

Schwartz D et al. (1989) Brain Res 482: 261.

Tecott LH et al. (1995) Nature 374: 542.

Tohyama IM et al. (1988) Neuroscience 26: 971.

Dexfenfluramine: Biological Regulator of Risk Factors for Overeating

John E. Blundell

BioPsychology Group, Department of Psychology, University of Leeds, Leeds LS2 9JT, UK

VULNERABILITY TO WEIGHT GAIN

It is becoming widely accepted that there is an asymmetrical regulation of body weight. Anthropological, epidemiological and experimental evidence suggests that it is easier for human beings to gain weight than to reduce weight. The body appears to generate strong physiological defences against a reduction of energy intake and weight loss but a much weaker resistance to weight gain. One factor contributing to weight gain is the increase in energy intake mediated through eating behaviour (Blundell, 1996). This overconsumption coupled with a permissive physiological system can therefore favour the development of a positive energy balance, which in turn will lead to weight gain and the maintenance of a high body mass index. There are compelling reasons why any treatment for obesity must confront the problem of overconsumption. It is of course recognized that a positive energy balance can be achieved via an increase in energy intake or a relative decrease in energy expenditure. Both of these aspects are important. However, because of the psychological importance of eating, the pleasure it provides, the powerful contingencies controlling eating habits and the potent attractiveness of the food supply, obese people will always have a problem to manage their energy intake. A drug which acts as a physiological regulator can provide biological assistance for this management. In particular an anti-obesity drug which operates, at least in part, by controlling energy intake must be capable of countering the risk factors for high energy intakes.

Obesity Management and Redux[TM]
ISBN 0-12-518170-1

RISK FACTORS FOR OVEREATING

It is possible to identify a number of risk factors which lead to increases in energy intake and which therefore favour the development of a positive energy balance. These risk factors include patterns of behaviour, physiological sensors and signals, sensory and nutritional features of the food supply, drives to eat and other subjective sensations.

Hunger and urges to eat. There is a good deal of evidence that the perceived intensity of hunger prior to an eating episode correlates well with the amount of food subsequently consumed. For example, when food intake and hunger were monitored for several days, subjective hunger was the best predictor of meal size and was negatively correlated with the energy value of stomach contents (de Castro and Elmore, 1988). Another study has reported a positive correlation of 0.5 between hunger and food intake at every hour across the day (Mattes, 1990). Under other circumstances such as nutritional loading, coefficients may be in the region of 0.6–0.75 (Hill and Blundell, 1990). Although the claim is often heard that obese people deny that hunger is a cause of their eating, when obese subjects are scientifically investigated there is normally a synchronous relationship between their experience of hunger and the amount of food consumed (Lawton *et al.*, 1993).

Nutrient composition: energy density and fat. There is good evidence that the nutrient composition of foods is a risk factor for overconsumption. The key variable appears to be energy density; individuals exposed to high energy density diets consume more energy than those eating low energy density foods (Weinsier *et al.*, 1982). The major contributor to energy density in foods is *dietary fat* and high fat diets invariably generate high levels of energy intake (Lissner *et al.*, 1987). This applies to obese (Lawton *et al.*, 1993) as well as lean individuals (Green *et al.*, 1994) when offered high-fat (low-carbohydrate) and low-fat (high-carbohydrate diets). A number of large-scale surveys have demonstrated a positive correlation between the percentage of fat in the diet and weight gain or body mass index (e.g. Dreon *et al.*, 1988).

Relatively weak satiety signals. The pattern of eating is largely influenced by processes occurring during consumption (satiation) and those which follow eating (post-ingestive satiety). There is mounting evidence that dietary fat exerts disproportionately weak post-ingestive inhibitory effects compared with carbohydrate or protein (Lawton *et al.*, 1993; Cotton *et al.*, 1994; Rolls *et al.*, 1994). Although, under experimental circumstances strong fat-induced physiological satiety signals can be detected (e.g. Welch *et al.*, 1985), they appear to be weaker than other nutrient-induced signals, at least in some vulnerable individuals. This issue has given rise to the 'fat paradox' which contrasts the presence of fat-related satiety signals with the hyperphagia readily demonstrable with high-fat diets (Blundell *et al.*, 1995). In this further way dietary fat constitutes a risk factor for overconsumption.

Palatability and sensory features of foods. In considering the capacity for energy intake to rise above expenditure, the weakness of inhibitory factors (e.g. certain satiety signals – see above) has to be set against the potency of facilitatory processes. The perceived pleasantness of food (palatability) is clearly one feature which could exert a positive influence over eating behaviour. This principle is well recognized by the food industry, which is ever seeking to enhance the sensory attractiveness of foods. Palatability does indeed influence the cumulative energy intake curve (Kissileff, 1984) and it can be deduced that the perceived palatability of particular foods by obese individuals puts them at risk of overconsumption (Drewnowski *et al.*, 1992). In addition, particular sensory and nutrient combinations, which produce potent hedonic responses, favour overconsumption (Green and Blundell, 1995). Obese people appear to perceive high-fat foods as being highly palatable. Palatability is therefore a further risk factor for overconsumption.

Craving for carbohydrates. There is a considerable body of evidence indicating a link between the ratio of protein to carbohydrate consumed and the access of trytophan to the brain (Wurtman *et al.*, 1982). This is believed to culminate in an increased synthesis of brain serotonin. In a number of conditions it is argued that certain individuals seek carbohydrate foods as a way of nutritionally adjusting their own neurochemistry and, in turn, improving their mood state. The high intake of carbohydrates (frequently accompanied by fat) may easily lead to a positive energy balance; therefore carbohydrate craving can be considered a risk factor for overconsumption.

Pattern of eating. It has generally been envisaged that two types of eating pattern favour overconsumption. These are a small number of very large meals, or a normal meal pattern with frequent snacks. Of course it is possible for any combination of meal size and number to yield an energy intake resulting in a positive energy balance. Probably the most important feature is the energy density of the foods consumed. However, large meals involving high-fat foods (with relatively weak post-ingestive satiety) and frequent snacks between meals (which do not significantly modulate hunger) appear to be high-risk eating patterns capable of producing overconsumption.

Mood and feelings of control. It is widely accepted that a negative mood state will promote eating (on the understanding that food acts as an antidepressant or an anxiolytic agent). Therefore, depressive or anxious states may constitute a risk factor for eating. In addition feelings of loss of control in the presence of food are typical of eating in binges and eating unconnected with nutritional requirements. Both of these categories of subjective states therefore may create a vulnerability to overconsumption.

It follows from this description of risk factors that an anti-obesity drug should adjust the regulatory system in such a way as to reduce the strength of these risk factors and to lessen their impact to generate a positive energy balance.

EFFECT OF DEXFENFLURAMINE ON OVERCONSUMPTION

Dexfenfluramine and energy intake

Initially it is necessary to demonstrate that dexfenfluramine can correct a positive energy balance, at least in part, by reducing energy intake. Those studies which have set out to monitor calorie consumption following the administration of dexfenfluramine demonstrate an unambiguous outcome. That is, all the studies currently under review have found clear and unequivocal reductions in energy intake as a result of drug treatment. The study details are described briefly in Table 1. The extent of the decrease in energy intake varies from study to study, but is apparent in treatment regimes ranging from a single day to 6 months. More importantly, the restraint exerted by dexfenfluramine over energy intake is evident even after 1 year of treatment. In the 12-month international multicentre trial the withdrawal of dexfenfluramine at the end of 1 year led to an immediate rise in daily energy consumed (Guy-Grand *et al.*, 1990). This indicates that the drug had continued to hold food intake in check and had effectively controlled the capacity of the risk factors to generate high energy intake.

Dexfenfluramine and dietary fat intake

It has been noted earlier that dietary fat is a potent risk factor for overconsumption. It is therefore important that an anti-obesity drug is able to oppose the stimulating effect of fat on energy intake. The analysis of animal studies demonstrates two features. First, exposure of rats to high levels of dietary fat (leading to hyperphagia and weight gain) does not impede the

Table 1
A summary of studies measuring the effects of dexfenfluramine on energy intake

Study	Subjects' weight	Dosing	Assessment	Change in energy intake
Silverstone et al. (1987)	Normal	1 day	Single test meal	↓ 40% test meal intake
Goodall and Silverstone (1988)	Normal	1 day	Single test (2 h)	↓ 25% test meal intake
Blundell and Hill (1988)	Normal	1 day	Single test meal	↓ 11% test meal intake
Hill and Blundell (1986)[a]	Normal	5 days	Single test meal; diary records	↓ 18% test meal intake
	Normal	5 days		↓ 25% total daily intake
Hill and Blundell (1990)[a]	Obese	3 days	Single test meal	↓ 11% test meal intake
Wurtman et al. (1985)	Obese (CHO cravers)	8 days	Measured meals and snacks	↓ 23% total daily intake
Wurtman et al. (1987)	Obese (CHO cravers)	3 months	Measured meals and snacks	↓ 22% total daily intake
	Obese (non-CHO cravers)	3 months	Measured meals and snacks	↓ 22% total daily intake
Andersen et al. (1989)	Obese	6 months	Diary records	↓ 13% total daily intake more than placebo

[a]15 mg on test day; all other studies 30 mg; CHO, carbohydrates.

suppressive effects of serotonergic agents on food intake or body weight. Indeed, dexfenfluramine appears to be particularly effective, and for long periods with very-high-fat diets. Second, in those circumstances where rats have been offered choices of diets including fat, serotonergic agents have demonstrated at least some suppression of fat choice, and in certain cases, a preferential suppression of fat intake. It is clear that dexfenfluramine administration is a sufficient stimulus to block the hyperphagia and antagonize the weight gain associated with high levels of dietary fat (Blundell and Lawton, 1995).

Interestingly, it has become clear that the action of dexfenfluramine on the eating pattern in humans will inevitably produce a major reduction in fat consumption. One prominent effect of dexfenfluramine is a reduction of snacking. As Drewnowski (1987) has pointed out, snack foods contain large amounts of fat (40–60%) and some snack items used in experiments contain as much as 81% fat. Therefore, any inhibitory action on the consumption of snack foods will induce an obligatory reduction in dietary fat, which normally makes the greatest contribution to energy of any single nutrient. This effect has been further demonstrated in a study on food intake in women with premenstrual depression (Brezinski et al., 1990). Foods available in the experimental unit varied in protein and CHO content but were consistently high in fat (45–60%). Items were designed to be iso-fat, and sometimes butter, cream or mayonnaise were used to increase the fat content. During the luteal phase, subjects showed an increased preference for CHO snacks (which contained large quantities of fat) and this tendency was antagonized in dexfenfluramine-treated subjects. Therefore, dexfenfluramine reduced CHO together with fat.

Even though dexfenfluramine potently reduces the intake of high-fat foods, it can be questioned whether serotonergic agents produce any *selective avoidance* or suppression of dietary fat intake. In a recent clinical study on obese subjects, further evidence has been provided for a selective action of dexfenfluramine on fat intake. Thirty obese subjects with a degree of excess weight of 20–80% of ideal weight were assigned to 3-month treatment periods on either placebo or dexfenfluramine (30 mg day^{-1}). The main focus of the study was an examination of basal metabolic rate and postprandial thermogenesis, but body weight and energy intakes were also monitored (Lafreniere et al., 1993). At the end of the 3-month treatment period, the measured energy intake of the dexfenfluramine group was 16% less than that of the placebo group. (Food intake was measured objectively for one complete day in the metabolic ward.) This consisted of a 13% reduction from meals and a 23% reduction from snacks. The energy reduction was characterized by a selective decrease in dietary lipids from 34% to 30% of total energy. By calculation, this represents a 25% reduction in the amount of fat consumed. Therefore, this result appears to show a selective avoidance of fat foods by subjects receiving dexfenfluramine.

Taken together, these human studies demonstrate that high-fat foods do not impede and may even strengthen the suppression of eating by dexfenfluramine. Whenever high-fat foods have been offered to subjects, dexfenfluramine has shown an effective reduction of intake. Moreover, there is also some evidence that administration (short-term or prolonged) of dexfenfluramine can induce a selective avoidance of high-fat foods and lead to an overall reduction in dietary lipids.

Table 2
Dexfenfluramine reduces the risk factors for overeating

Risk factor	Effect of dexfenfluramine	Reference
Urge to eat	Reduced strength of urges	Hill *et al.* (1995)
Inter-meal motivation to eat	Suppression of desire to eat between meals	Blundell and Hill (1987)
Intensity of hunger	Decreased	Goodall and Silverstone (1988)
Large meal size	Reduced intake with buffet meals	Hill and Blundell (1986)
Snacking frequency	Reduced	Wurtman *et al.* (1985)
High-fat foods (acute)	Greater reduction of fat than other macronutrients	Goodall *et al.* (1993)
Dietary fat (long-term)	Selective reduction (25% decrease)	Lafreniere *et al.* (1993)
Weak post-ingestive satiety	Increased satiating action of food	Blundell and Hill (1989)
Carbohydrate craving	Reduction of carbohydrate (and fat) during phases of craving	Brezinski *et al.* (1990)
Low mood and loss of control	Improved mood and increased feeling of control over eating	Hill *et al.* (1995)
Potent hedonic food qualities (high palatability, high energy density)	Suppressed intake of foods with strong sensory attractiveness	Wurtman *et al.* (1987)

DEXFENFLURAMINE AND THE RISK FACTORS FOR OVEREATING

Many human beings, probably a majority, demonstrate a vulnerability to gain weight. One reason for this is the apparent ease with which certain people allow the development of a positive energy balance. The risk factors which provoke the occurrence of a positive energy balance reside within the biological system, in the environment (in the food supply itself) and at the interface between food and the biological system. Some of the most potent risk factors which generate unwanted overconsumption (energy intake rising above energy expenditure) have been described above.

Research which has accumulated over the course of more than a decade indicates that dexfenfluramine significantly reduces all of the major risk factors for overeating (see Table 2). It follows that if dexfenfluramine is an antagonist of the risk factors then one consequence will be a reduced level of energy intake. The evidence shows that dexfenfluramine has the capacity to inhibit consumption even in the face of potent risk factors such as strong urges to eat, high levels of hunger, the presence of high-fat foods and the presence of high-palatability foods with powerful hedonic qualities. Some of the internalized risk factors such as hunger, carbohydrate seeking, urges to eat and weak satiety signals can be considered as psychobiological markers of overconsumption. Factors concerning the eating pattern (large meals, binges, or increased tendency to snack) can be considered as behavioural markers, and factors in the food supply such as high-fat, high-palatability foods (stimulating sensory-nutrient combinations) can be considered environmental markers of overeating. It is therefore important that the action of dexfenfluramine, mediated via serotoninergic processes, is effective against the psychobiological, behavioural and environmental markers of overconsumption.

RISK FACTORS AND WEIGHT GAIN: SUMMARY

Many people are vulnerable to weight gain because of a permissive physiological system in the presence of a potent and stimulating food supply in a provocative environment. This combination appears to lead rather easily to a positive energy balance. A number of risk factors for overconsumption have been identified. Experimental and clinical evidence indicates that dexfenfluramine effectively reduces the potency of these risk factors (urges to eat, energy dense foods, high levels of dietary fat, hunger, large meals and frequent snacks, strong sensory attractiveness of foods, loss of control and relatively weak satiety signals), and thereby lessens their impact on energy intake. Obese people find it extremely difficult (usually impossible) to prevent themselves drifting into positive energy balance through involuntary (passive) overconsumption and sometimes through active food seeking. Significantly, this drug is clearly effective in inhibiting the intake of some of the most palatable and sensorily attractive foods that the food industry can manufacture. Dexfenfluramine can provide biological assistance to allow obese people to control those risk factors for weight gain operating via overconsumption.

REFERENCES

Anderson A, Astrup A, Quaade F (1989) d-Fenfluramine reduces overweight but does not change food preferences. *Int J Obesity* **13** (suppl. 1): 136.

Blundell JE (1996) Food intake and body weight regulation. In: Bouchard C and Bray GA (eds) *Regulation of Body Weight: Biological and Behavioral Mechanisms*. John Wiley & Sons Ltd, London: 111–133.

Blundell JE, Hill AJ (1987) Serotoninergic modulation of the pattern of eating and the profile of hunger-satiety in humans. *Int J Obesity* **11** (suppl. 3): 141–155.

Blundell JE, Hill AJ (1988) On the mechanism of action of dexfenfluramine: Effect on alliesthesia and appetite motivation in lean and obese subjects. *Clin Pharmacol* **11** (suppl. 1): S121–S134.

Blundell JE, Hill AJ (1989) Serotoninergic drug potentiates the satiating capacity of food: Action of d-fenfluramine in obese subjects. *Ann NY Acad Sci* **575**: 493–495.

Blundell JE, Lawton CL (1995) Serotonin and dietary fat intake: Effects of dexfenfluramine. *Metabolism* **44**(2): 33–37.

Blundell JE, Burley VJ, Cotton JR et al. (1995) The fat paradox: Fat-induced satiety signals but overconsumption on high fat foods. *Int J Obesity* **19**: 832–835.

Brezinski AA, Wurtman JJ, Wurtman RJ (1990) D-fenfluramine suppresses the increased caloric and carbohydrate intakes and improves the mood of women with pre-menstrual tension. *Obstet Gynecol* **76**: 296–301.

Cotton JR, Burley VJ, Weststrate JA, Blundell JE (1994) Dietary fat and appetite: Similarities and differences in the satiating effect of meals supplemented with either fat and/or carbohydrate. *J Hum Nutr Diet* **7**: 11–24.

de Castro JM, Elmore DK (1988) Subjective hunger relationships with meal patterns in the spontaneous feeding behaviour of humans: Evidence for a causal connection. *Physiol Behav* **43**: 159–165.

Dreon DM, Frey-Hewitt B, Ellsworth N et al. (1988) Dietary fat: Carbohydrate ratio and obesity in middle aged men. *Am J Clin Nutr* **47**: 995–1000.

Drewnowski A (1987) Changes in mood after carbohydrate consumption. *Am J Clin Nutr* **46**: 703.

Drewnowski A, Kurth C, Holden-Wiltse J, Saari J (1992) Food preferences in human obesity: Carbohydrates versus fats. *Appetite* **18**: 207–221.

Goodall E, Silverstone JT (1988) Different effect of d-fenfluramine and metergoline on food intake in human subjects. *Appetite* **11**: 215–228.

Goodall EM, Cowen PJ, Franklin M (1993) Ritanserin attenuates anorectic, endocrine and thermic responses to D-fenfluramine in human volunteers. *Psychopharmacology* **112**: 461–466.

Green S, Blundell JE (1995) Capacity of high sucrose and high fat foods to satisfy hunger in lean dietary unrestrained and restrained females. *Int J Obesity* **19** (suppl. 2): 79.

Green S, Burley VJ, Blundell JE (1994) Effect of fat-containing and sucrose-containing foods on the size of eating episodes and energy intake in lean males: Potential for causing overconsumption. *Eur J Clin Nutr* **48**: 547–555.

Guy-Grand B, Apfelbaum M, Crepaldi G et al. (1990) Effect of withdrawal of dexfenfluramine on body weight and food intake after a one year's administration. *Int J Obesity* **14** (suppl. 2): 48.

Hill AJ, Blundell JE (1986) Model system for investigating the actions of anorectic drugs: Effect of D-fenfluramine on food intake, nutrient selection, food preferences, meal patterns, hunger and satiety in healthy human subjects. *Adv Biosci* **60**: 377–389.

Hill AJ, Blundell JE (1990) Sensitivity of the appetite control system in obese subjects to nutritional and serotoninergic challenges. *Int J Obesity* **14**: 219–233.

Hill AJ, Lawton CL, Wales JK, Blundell JE (1995) Dexfenfluramine and the control of eating: Effects on obese women living at home. *Int J Obesity* **19** (suppl. 2): 142.

Kissileff HR (1984) Satiating efficiency and a strategy for conducting food loading experiments. *Neuroscio Biobehav Rev* **8**: 129–135.

Lafreniere F, Lambert J, Rasio E (1993) Effects of dexfenfluramine treatment on body weight and postprandial thermogenesis in obese subjects. A double-blind placebo-controlled study. *Int J Obesity* **17**: 25–30.

Lawton CL, Burley VJ, Wales JK, Blundell JE (1993) Dietary fat and appetite control in obese subjects: Weak effects on satiation and satiety. *Int J Obesity* **17**: 409–416.

Lissner L, Levitsky DA, Strupp BJ et al. (1987) Dietary fat and the regulation of energy intake in human subjects. *Am J Clin Nutr* **46**: 886–892.

Mattes R (1990) Hunger ratings are not a valid proxy measure of reported food intakes in humans. *Appetite* **15**: 103–113.

Rolls BJ, Kim-Harris S, Fischman MW et al. (1994) Satiety after preloads with different amounts of fat and carbohydrate: Implications for obesity. *Am J Clin Nutr* **60**: 476–487.

Silverstone T, Smith G, Richards R (1987) A comparative evaluation of dexfenfluramine and dl-fenfluramine on hunger, food intake, psychomotor function and side effects in normal human subjects. In: Bender AE and Brooks LJ (eds) *Body Weight Control. The Physiology, Clinical Treatment and Prevention of Obesity.* Churchill Livingstone, London: 240–246.

Weinsier RC, Johnston MH, Doleys DM, Bacon JA (1982) Dietary management of obesity: Evaluation of the time–energy displacement diet in terms of its efficacy and nutritional adequacy for long-term weight control. *Br J Nutr* **47**: 367–379.

Welch I, Saunders K, Read NW (1985) Effect of ileal and intravenous infusions of fat emulsions on feeding and satiety in human volunteers. *Gastroenterology* **89**: 1293–1297.

Wurtman JJ, Wurtman RJ, Growdon JH (1982) Carbohydrate craving in obese people: suppression by treatments affecting serotoninergic transmission. *Int J Eating Disord* **1**: 2–15.

Wurtman J, Wurtman R, Marks S et al. (1985) D-Fenfluramine selectively suppresses carbohydrate snacking by obese subjects. *Int J Eating Dis* **4**: 89–99.

Wurtman J, Wurtman R, Reynolds S et al. (1987) Fenfluramine suppresses snack intake among carbohydrate cravers but not among noncarbohydrate cravers. *Int J Eating Dis* **6**: 687–699.

Part II

Methods for Assessing Neurochemical Changes and their Effect

Advancement of Knowledge on Fenfluramine and Dexfenfluramine Effects on Brain Chemistry

Madhu Kalia

Professor of Neurosurgery, Jefferson Medical College, Thomas Jefferson University, Philadelphia, PA 19107, USA

INTRODUCTION

Since 1976 over 600 full-length papers, rapid communications, letters to editors and abstracts have appeared in the literature on the subject of fenfluramine and/or dexfenfluramine-induced neurochemical changes. The purpose of this review is not to provide the reader with a comprehensive discussion of these publications, but rather to provide a historical perspective of the subject of dexfenfluramine-induced neurochemical changes with a specific focus on the question of whether dexfenfluramine produces pathological changes in the cell bodies and nerve terminals of serotoninergic neurons in the brainstem. An extensive review of all the pertinent data has revealed that there is no evidence to indicate that dexfenfluramine produces neurotoxic changes in these neurons.

The issue of fenfluramine-induced neurotoxicity was first raised by Harvey and McMaster (1975, 1977) and Harvey *et al.* (1977). These investigators reported changes in neurons within brainstem nuclei known to contain serotoninergic neurons.

ROBBINS' STUDIES

Following these initial studies, the manufacturer of fenfluramine tablets, A.H. Robbins, conducted three complete histological studies using single doses of fenfluramine ranging from 1.0 to 31.6 mg kg^{-1} and sacrifice times of 72 h and

Obesity Management and Redux^{TM}
ISBN 0-12-518170-1

30 days. Other drugs and saline were used as controls. Recommended histological techniques furnished by Harvey were used in preparing the histological slides. Three pathologists, including a neuropathologist, examined the slides. Hyperchromic, misshaped (dark) neurons and perineural spaces were found in areas B7, B8 and B9 as reported by Harvey and McMaster (1975). However, these neurons were also found in the non-serotoninergic neurons in the mesencephalic nucleus of the fifth nerve, the third nerve nucleus, the lateral midbrain reticular formation and the pontine nuclei. The same changes were found in the controls as well as in animals treated with reference drugs, p-chloramphetamine and reserpine. The three pathologists concluded that the changes found in all groups of animals were artifactual (Funderburk, 1977).

FDA ADVISORY COMMITTEE MEETING ON 13 JUNE 1978

The specific issue of whether fenfluramine produced pathological changes in brainstem neurons was reviewed at a meeting of the FDA's Peripheral and CNS Drugs Advisory Committee on 13 June 1978. The following summary of the presentations made at that meeting highlights the information about the issue available at that time.

The meeting began with a review of Dr Harvey's work, the major findings of which are noted above. Following Dr Harvey's presentation, Dr Steve Hendrickson presented results from his laboratory. In his initial study, he used a specific fluorescence histochemical technique to demonstrate serotonin neurons after fenfluramine administration. With administration of 20 mg kg^{-1} of fenfluramine for 4 days and sacrifice of animals 1 month later, Dr Hendrickson found no significant decrease in serotonin neurons in the raphe nuclei in the treated animals when compared with controls. Indeed, the fenfluramine-treated animals had a slightly greater number of serotonin neurons. Dr Hendrickson also presented data from brains prepared with a silver stain, one of the methods used by Dr Harvey, but was unable to find pathological changes.

An independent study done by Hazelton Laboratories also failed to confirm the findings reported by Harvey.

Dr Robert Moore reported a study in which he used two different paradigms. In the first, he repeated Dr Harvey's paradigm exactly and, in the second, he repeated the treatment paradigm but used a separate, and more appropriate, method of fixation. The first study produced data essentially identical to Dr Harvey's, but the second, using optimal fixation, showed no difference between fenfluramine-treated animals and controls. Dr Moore concluded that the pyknotic changes in Dr Harvey's material were not pathological but represented an interaction between a functional neuronal event and suboptimal fixation.

Dr Constantino Sotelo reviewed material from his laboratory and found no clear abnormality at either the light of electron microscopic level.

Dr Kenneth Earle, Director of Neuropathology at the Armed Forces Institute of Pathology, reported on his review of Dr Harvey's material and other materials supplied by the A.H. Robbins Co., and stated that he observed the same changes reported by Dr Harvey but concluded that there was no evidence of any neuropathology induced by fenfluramine.

On the basis of these presentations, the FDA Advisory Committee concluded that there was no substantive evidence that fenfluramine produced pathological changes in brainstem neurons and that there was no basis for further action. While doing so, however, the FDA Advisory Committee encouraged further investigations.

RESULTS OF POST-1978 STUDIES

Basic Neuroanatomy of Serotoninergic Neurons in the Raphe Nuclei

The cell bodies of most serotoninergic neurons in the brain are located largely within the midline raphe nuclei (Dahlstrom and Fuxe, 1964) and project directly to most areas of the brain and spinal cord (Fuxe, 1965; Anden et al., 1966; Azmitia and Segal, 1978). The 5-HT innervation of the cerebral cortex arises primarily from the rostral-most raphe nuclei, located in the mesencephalon, the dorsal raphe (DR), median raphe (MR) and the D9 cell groups (Conrad et al., 1974; Bobillier et al., 1975; Azmitia and Segal, 1978; Jacobs et al., 1978; Moore et al., 1978; Parent et al., 1981; Kohler and Steinbusch, 1982; Galindo-Mireles et al., 1985). While the B9 cell group is not well characterized, the dorsal and median raphe form two distinct sets of 5-HT neurons with dissimilar projections. These nuclei give rise to separate ascending fibre bundles (Azmitia and Segal, 1978) and preferentially innervate different forebrain regions (Lorens and Goldberg, 1974; Bobillier et al., 1975; Azmitia and Segal, 1978; Jacobs et al., 1978; Kohler et al., 1980).

Results of Light Microscopy Studies since 1978

Studies with light microscopy have not indicated any cell loss or aberration in nerve networks. The results of such studies are summarized below.

Sotelo and Zamora (1979) gave rats 100 μmol kg^{-1} (27 mg kg^{-1}) of fenfluramine and examined two populations of neurons in the B9 cell group after survival times ranging from 1 to 30 days. Nissl staining and the Fink Heimer technique were used to examine the morphological changes at the light microscopic level. Neither perineuronal spaces nor hyperchromic dark neurons were observed. In addition, no degenerating neuronal perikarya or dendrites were observed, nor were any changes observed at the ultrastructural level. Similarly, Lorez *et al.* (1978) failed to find any changes in the B6 group.

There is increasing evidence that 'cell bodies of 5-HT neurons in the raphe nuclei do not show changes after fenfluramine treatment' (Molliver and Molliver, 1990). Four-day fenfluramine treatment did not appear to affect serotoninergic cell bodies in the various raphe nuclei (Appel *et al.*, 1989). Serotonin-like immunostained cell bodies from treated animals were unremarkable in appearance and displayed normal morphology and staining intensity similar to that seen in saline-injected rats (Appel *et al.*, 1989). Although cell counts were not performed by Molliver and Molliver, it did not appear that the number of stained cell bodies differed significantly between the treated and control groups (Molliver and Molliver, 1990).

It should be pointed out that these studies have employed the use of a polyclonal antibody directed 5-HT, which has permitted the visualization of 5-HT perikarya (cell bodies) as well as terminals. By using such a specific technique the question of whether 5-HT raphe neurons are damaged by fenfluramine has been resolved, and no evidence of neuronal damage has been found (Appel *et al.*, 1989; Molliver and Molliver, 1990).

In one study there is particularly persuasive evidence of the lack of morphological changes in raphe serotoninergic neurons (Molliver and Molliver, 1990). In this study immunocytochemical staining was utilized to 'assess anatomic evidence of an acute effect of fenfluramine upon serotoninergic neurons, to determine whether the drug has lasting neurotoxic effects, and to identify specific neurons and neuronal processes that may be damaged'. The experiments showed a 'marked decrease in the number of 5-HT immunoreactive axons throughout the forebrain'. The experiments also showed 'that axons of passage and cell bodies of origin are spared after fenfluramine administration'.

Results of Studies using Axonal Transport as an Index of Functional Integrity

The functional viability of the 5-HT neurons in the raphe nuclei, including their cortical nerve terminal networks, was tested using a retrograde transport label (cholera-toxin conjugated with horseradish peroxidase, CTHRP) in rats treated with dexfenfluramine or a positive control (*p*-chloramphetamine,

PCA), a known serotonin neurotoxin (Kalia and O'Malley, 1993). The goal of this study was to examine the effect of different doses of dexfenfluramine on the functional viability of brain serotoninergic neurons. Disruption of axonal transport in the raphe–cortical serotoninergic system has been as a primary indicator of neuronal injury (Mamounas and Molliver, 1988).

The functional viability of the raphe–cortical serotoninergic system was described by injection of CTHRP into the cortex and examining the midbrain dorsal and median raphe nuclei for the presence of retrogradely transported CTHRP. This method enabled Kalia *et al.* to test for two systems: (1) the viability of the 5-HT nerve terminals in the cortex as measured by their ability to take up CTHRP, and (2) the viability of the 5-HT perikarya in the dorsal raphe nucleus as measured by their ability to accumulate the CTHRP as a result of retrograde transport.

The total number of serotoninergic raphe neurons retrogradely labelled with a standardized volume of the tracer CTHRP injected in the cortical terminal fields was counted in serial sections in dexfenfluramine-treated, PCA-treated and pair-fed controls (Kalia and O'Malley, 1993). The number of serotoninergic raphe neurons retrogradely labelled in PCA-treated animals was significantly lower (66%) than in pair-fed controls. Dexfenfluramine-treated animals showed no reduction in the number of retrogradely labelled serotoninergic neurons as compared with pair-fed controls. This demonstrates that axonal transport is not impaired by dexfenfluramine. This finding is consistent with earlier studies using similar dexfenfluramine-treatment proto-cols and using the serotonin immunocytochemistry of raphe neurons.

Results of Ultrastructural Studies since 1978

Olivier *et al.* (1978) attempted to reproduce the possible toxic effect of fenfluramine in 5-HT cells on B8 and B9 areas. Olivier *et al.* injected i.p. $100\,\mu\text{mol kg}^{-1}$ (27 mg kg^{-1}) of fenfluramine or saline. One, 3 or 10 days after fenfluramine treatment. No degenerative changes were found with any survival period despite the decrease of brain 5-HT content. Increasing the fenfluramine doses from 5 to 200 μmol kg^{-1} in 10 days showed no neuronal abnormality or glial reaction in the brains of rats sacrificed 24 h after the last administration.

CONCLUSION

Since the original reports by Drs Harvey and McMaster of perikaryal changes in neurons of brainstem serotoninergic nuclei (1975, 1977) there have been a number of studies that have addressed this issue. Without exception, even at doses as high as 48 mg kg^{-1} day^{-1} of dexfenfluramine, studies have failed to find any evidence of perikaryal changes after dexfenfluramine administration. Furthermore, studies of retrograde transport, which depends upon the functional integrity of the serotonin neurons, do not show any indication of functional impairment. Finally, reviews of the material from the original study by Drs Harvey and McMaster and replications of the study in several laboratories have been interpreted as not showing neuropathological changes. Consequently, it is concluded that fenfluramine does not produce pathological changes and cell loss in serotoninergic neurons of the brainstem raphe.

REFERENCES

Anden NE, Dahlstrom A, Fuxe K, Larsson K, Olson L and Ungerstedt U (1966) Ascending monoamine neurons to the telecephalon and diencephalon. *Acta. Physiol. Scand.* **87**: 313–316.

Appel NM, Contrera JF and De Souza EB (1989) Fenfluramine selectively and differentially decreases the dendity of serotonergic nerve terminals in rat brain: evidence from immunocytochemical studies. *J. Pharmacol. Exp. Ther.* **245**: 928–943.

Azmitia EC and Segal M (1978) An autoradiographic analysis of the differential ascending projections of the dorsal and median raphe nuclei in the rat. *J. Comp. Neurol.* **167**: 641–668.

Bobillier P, Sequin S, Petitjean F, Salvert D, Touret M and Jouvet M (1976) The raphe nuclei of the cat brain stem. A topographical atlas of their efferent projections as revealed by autoradiography. *Brain Res.* **113**: 449–486.

Conrad L, Leonard C and Pfaffi S. (1974) Connections of the median and dorsal raphe nuclei in the rat: An autoradiographic and degeneration study. *J. Comp. Neurol.* **156**: 176–206.

Dahlstrom A and Fuxe K (1964) Evidence for the existence of monoamine neurons. I. Demonstration of monoamines in cell bodies of brian neurons. *Acta. Physiol. Scand.* **63**, supp. 232, 1–55.

Funderburk FR In: Transcript of the June 18th FDA Advisory Committee Meeting (1978).

Fuxe K (1965). Evidence for the existence of monoamine neurons. IV. Distribution of monoamine nerve terminals in the central nervous system. *Acta Physiol. Scand. suppl.* **247**: 37–85.

Galindo-Mireles D, Myer A, Casteneyra-Perdomo A and Ferres-Torres R (1985) Cortical projections of the nucleus centralis superior and the adjacent reticular formation in the mouse. *Brain Res.* **330**: 343–348.

Harvey J and McMaster SE (1975) Fenfluramine: Evidence for a neurotoxic action on midbrain and a long-term depletion of serotonin. *Psychopharmacol. Commun.* **1**: 217–228.

Harvey JA and McMaster SE (1977) Cumulative neurotoxicity after chronic treatment with low dosages in the rat. *Comm. in Psychopharmacology* **1**: 3–17.

Harvey JA, McMaster SE and Fuller RW (1977) Comparison between the neurotoxic and serotonin-depleting effects of various halogenated derivatives of amphetamine in the rat. *J. Pharmacol. Exp. Ther.* **202**: 581–589.

Jacobs BL, Foote SL and Bloom FE (1978) Differential projections of neurons within the dorsal raphe nucleus of the rat: *A horseradish peroxidase (HRP) study*. *Brain Res*. **147**: 149–153.

Kalia M and O'Malley NP (1993) Brain serotonergic neurons demonstrate normal axonal transport following short and long-term treatment with dexfenfluramine. *Soc. Neurosc. Abstr.* **19**: 1060.

Kohler K and Steinbusch HWM (1982) Identification of serotonin and non-serotonin containing neurons of the mid-brain raphe projections to the entominal area of the hippocampal formation. A combined immunocytochemical and fluorescent retrograde tracing study in the rat brain. *Neuroscience* **7**: 951–970.

Lorens SA and Goldberg HC (1974) Regional 5-hydroxytryptamine following selective midbrain raphe lesions in the rat. *Brain Res*. **78**: 45–56.

Lorez HP, Saner A and Richards JG (1978) Evidence agains a neurotoxic action of halogenated amphetamines on serotonergic B9 cells. *Brain Res*. **146**: 188–194.

Mamounas LA and Molliver ME (1988) Dual serotonergic projections to forebrain have separate origins in the dorsal and median raphe nuclei: retrograde transport after selective ablation by *p*-chloroamphetamine (PCA). *Soc. Neurosc. Abstr.* **13**: 907.

Molliver DC and Molliver ME (1990) Anatomical evidence for a neurotoxic effect of fenfluramine upon serotonergic projections in the rat. *Brain Res*. **511**: 165–168.

Moore RY, Halaris AE and Jones BE (1978) Serotonin neurons of the mid-brain raphe: ascending projections. *J. Comp. Neurol*. **180**: 417–438.

Olivier L, dr Boistesselin R and Duhault J (1978) Lack of histological neurotoxicity during fenfluramine treatment in the rat. *IRCS Medical Science* **6**: 463.

Parent A, Descarries L and Beaudet A (1981) Organization of ascending serotonin neurons in the adult rat brain. A radioautographic study after intraventricular administration of [^{3}H] 5-Hydroxytryptamine. *Neuroscience* **6**: 115–138.

Stoleo C and Zamora A (1979) Lack of morphological changes in neurons of B-9 group in rats treated with fenfluramine. *Curr. Med. Res. Opin.* **6** Suppl. 1 55–62.

Reactive Gliosis as an Indicator of Neurotoxicity

James P. O'Callaghan

*Neurotoxicology Division, National Health and Environmental Effects
Research Laboratory, US Environmental Protection Agency, Research
Triangle Park, NC 27711, USA*

Diverse types of injury to the central nervous system result in hypertrophy of astrocytes, a subtype of central nervous system glia. The hallmark of this response, often termed 'reactive gliosis', is the enhanced expression of the major intermediate filament protein of astrocytes, glial fibrillary acidic protein (GFAP) (Miller and O'Callaghan, 1994; Norton *et al.*, 1992). These morphological observations suggest that GFAP may be a useful biochemical indicator of neurotoxicity. To investigate this possibility we have administered prototype neurotoxicants to experimental animals and then assessed the effects of these agents on the tissue content of GFAP, as determined by immunoassay. We found that assays of GFAP reveal dose-, time- and region-dependent patterns of neural injury, often at toxicant dosages below those that result in light microscopic evidence of cell loss or damage. No false positives have been seen following exposure to a variety of pharmacological agents. In rodent studies, measurement of GFAP has proven useful for distinguishing neurotoxic amphetamines, such as methamphetamine and methylenedioxymethamphetamine (MDMA), from non-neurotoxic non-amphetaminic anorectic agents, such as dexfenfluramine (O'Callaghan and Miller 1994; O'Callaghan *et al.*, 1995).

The mammalian central nervous system (CNS) is composed of a large and diverse array of its two principal cell types, neurons and glia. Given this extreme cellular heterogeneity, it is not surprising that different chemical insults to the CNS damage different regional, cellular and subcellular targets.

For most chemicals (including drugs) there often is no *a priori* basis for predicting which targets are damaged by a particular agent. The traditional solution to this dilemma has been to rely on standard histopathological stains to reveal sites of neural damage. While this approach is sufficient to reveal damage to neural perikarya arranged in readily identifiable nuclei or cell layers (e.g. in cerebellum or hippocampus), damage to diffuse populations of cells may escape detection. Moreover, traditional stains cannot reveal damage to subcellular elements of neurons (e.g. axons or synaptic terminals) or subcellular elements of oligodendroglia (e.g. the myelin sheath). Thus, there is a clear need for a more sensitive indicator of neurotoxicity that will reveal damage to any target, regardless of its regional, cellular or subcellular localization.

Just as there is a need to prevent false negatives in assessments of chemical and drug-induced neurotoxicity, there also is a need to prevent false positives. Any widely applicable approach to neurotoxicity assessment should serve to differentiate pharmacological effects of a drug or chemical in questions from toxicological effects, i.e. those associated with damage to the nervous system. This has become more of a problem in recent years owing to the tendency to view neurotoxicological effects as an extension of the pharmacological effects of the chemical or drug in question. For example, pesticides developed to inhibit cholinesterase often are deemed 'neurotoxic' if they are found to inhibit CNS cholinesterase, the effect that the compound was designed to achieve. Likewise, the decrease in brain serotonin that results from high-dose treatment of rodents with dexfenfluramine is viewed by some as a 'neurotoxic' response, even though such an effect is the predictable result of the drug's action to release serotonin from nerve terminals. Of course, chemical- and drug-induced alterations in endpoints associated with their known pharmacology may also be associated with nervous system damage. What is needed, therefore, is an indicator that will distinguish between neuropharmacological effects and neurotoxicological effects.

For at least a century, the neuropathology literature has documented that central nervous system injury results in hypertrophy and proliferation of astrocytes. This reponse, termed astrogliosis or reactive gliosis, is characterized at the electron microscopic level by the accumulation of glial filaments. A major constituent of these filaments subsequently was found to be a protein denoted glial fibrillary acidic protein. Antibodies to GFAP have been widely applied to document, qualitatively, the astrocyte reaction to a variety of disease and lesion-induced injuries of the CNS (Miller and O'Callaghan, 1994; Norton et al., 1992). In aggregate, these anatomical observations suggested that GFAP represents an ideal candidate for a general indicator of neurotoxicity, one that is potentially sensitive enough to detect all types of damage, yet specific enough to distinguish chemical- and drug-induced neural damage from pharmacological effects (Norton et al., 1992). To investigate this possibility, our strategy was to administer prototype neurotoxicants to experi-

Table 1
Prototype neurotoxicants and their known targets

Chemical/drug	Regional target	Cellular target	Subcellular target
Trimethyltin	Limbic structures	Neurons	Perikarya
Triethyltin	Myelinated structures	Oligodendroglia	Myelin sheath
Kainate	Limbic structures	Neurons	Perikarya
Bilirubin	Cerebellum	Purkinje cells	Perikarya
MPTP	Basal ganglia	Dopaminergic neurons	Nerve terminal
Cadmium	Basal ganglia	Neurons, glia?	?
Colchicine	Hippocampus	Granule cells	Microtubules
IDPN	Brainstem	Neurons	Neurofilaments
3-Acetyl pyridine	Inferior olive	Neurons	Perikarya
6-OHDA	Nigra/basal ganglia	Dopaminergic neurons	Perikarya/terminals
Methamphetamine	Basal ganglia	Dopaminergic neurons	Nerve terminal
5,7-DHT	Cortex, basal ganglia, hippocampus	Serotonergic neurons	Perikarya/terminals

MPTP = 1-methyl-4-phenyl-1,2,3,6-tetrahydropyridine; IDPN = iminodinitropropionitrile; 6-OHDA = 6-hydroxydopamine; 5,7-DHT = 5,7-dihydroxytryptamine. All targets refer to those known to be damaged by systemic or intracerebroventricular administration of the compound in question.

mental animals and quantify the effects of these agents on the tissue content of GFAP as assessed by immunoassay.

The hypothesis underlying the use of GFAP in neurotoxicity assessments was that homogenates of brain regions damaged by neurotoxic chemicals would contain increased levels of this protein (Norton *et al.*, 1992). To test this hypothesis, we have evaluated the effects of a number of prototype neurotoxicants and a variety of non-chemical brain insults on the regional levels of GFAP (Norton *et al.*, 1992). For the purpose of these validation studies, we defined a prototype neurotoxicant as any insult capable of causing damage to the cytoarchitecture of the nervous system as assessed by morphological criteria at the light microscopic or electron microscopic level. Examples of prototype neurotoxicants employed in our studies are listed in Table 1.

In selecting prototype neurotoxic insults, we purposely included toxicants or conditions that ranged from those causing overt cell loss to those that did not result in evidence of cell damage or loss based on traditional Nissl stains. By so doing, we could start our validation studies with compounds or conditions that were obviously neurotoxic, i.e. those that resulted in readily apparent neuron loss. We could then proceed to an examination of toxicants where verification of neurotoxicity would be more difficult, i.e. conditions where damage to specific cell types was not manifested by apparent neuropathological changes based on Nissl staining. The rationale for this validation scheme was straight-forward: prototype toxicants that would easily be detected by classical neuropathology screens must also produce substantial increases in GFAP. Otherwise, the GFAP-based approach, although quantitative, would not represent a major advance over current neuropathological evaluations. Like-wise, toxicants known to damage specific cell types without causing overt cytopathology also must show a positive GFAP response if the approach was to be successfully applied to screening neurotoxic compounds likely to be found in 'real world' scenarios. As part of our overall approach, we searched for potential false positive increases in GFAP by analysing brains obtained from rodents that had received therapeutic dosages of drugs known to affect a variety of CNS transmitter systems (Norton et al., 1992).

Three major conclusions that emerged from studies are as follows:

(1) *Assays of GFAP provide a* sensitive *means for assessing neurotoxicity*. All of the prototype neurotoxicants listed in Table 1 resulted in an increase in GFAP. As expected, compounds that resulted in overt cell loss, such as trimethyltin, caused large increases in GFAP. However, dosages of these compounds below those necessary to cause evidence for neuronal loss based on Nissl staining still resulted in an increase in GFAP. Thus, assays of GFAP were sensitive enough to reveal underlying damage in the absence of cytopathology. Moreover, prototype neurotoxicants that do not cause evidence of cytopathology based on Nissl staining, such as MPTP, still caused large dose-dependent increases in GFAP.

(2) *Increases in GFAP are* specific *to the neurotoxic state*. No false positives were seen using therapeutic dosage levels of drugs known to affect a variety of CNS systems. These include, for example, reserpine, pheno-barbital, diethylether, pargyline, apomorphine, morphine, scopolamine, atropine, parachlorophenylalanine, indomethacin, acetyl salicylic acid and fluoxetine.

(3) *Increases in GFAP can* differentiate *long-term neurochemical changes from neurotoxic effects*. For example, the administration of high, multiple-dose regimens of fenfluramine or dexfenfluramine to rats or mice results in a slowly reversible decrease in brain serotonin (O'Callaghan and Miller, 1994). These protracted neurochemical effects are not associated with an increase in GFAP (O'Callaghan and Miller, 1994). In contrast, a variety of amphetamines known to act on dopamine and serotonin neurons and the known serotonergic neurotoxicant, 5,7-dihydroxytryptamine, all produce large dose-related increases in GFAP in target appropriate brain regions (Norton et al., 1992; O'Callaghan and Miller, 1994; O'Callaghan et al., 1995). These data indicate that enhanced expression of GFAP can

be used to differentiate compounds that damage serotonergic and dopaminergic neurons from those that only reduce the levels of transmitter within
these neurons.

In summary, assays of GFAP represent one approach for neurotoxicity
assessment that can be used to differentiate pharmacological from neurotoxicological responses. Ideally, GFAP assays should be used in conjunction with
other general indicators of nervous system damage to offer the greatest
probability for detection of chemical- or drug-induced damage to any neural
element of the CNS.

REFERENCES

Miller DB, O'Callaghan JP (1994) Environment-, stress- and drug-induced alterations
    in body temperature affect the neurotoxicity of substituted amphetamines in the
    C57/B16J mouse. *J Pharmacol Exp Ther* **270**: 752–760.
Norton WT, Aquino DA, Hozumi I, Chiu F-C, Brosnan CF (1992) Quantitative
    aspects of reactive gliosis: A review. *Neurochem Res* **17**: 877–885.
O'Callaghan JP, Miller DB (1994) Neurotoxicity profiles of substituted amphetamines
    in the C57/B16J mouse. *J Pharmacol Exp Ther* **270**: 741–751.
O'Callaghan JP, Jensen KF, Miller DB (1995) Quantitative aspects of drug and
    toxicant-induced astrogliosis. *Neurochem Int* **26**: 115–124.

Dexfenfluramine Effects on Serotonin Neurons: A Long-term Immunohistochemical Analysis

Robert Y. Moore

Departments of Psychiatry, Neurology and Neuroscience, Center for Neuroscience, University of Pittsburgh, Pittsburgh, PA 15261, USA

INTRODUCTION

Serotonin (5-hydroxytryptamine, 5-HT) is produced by a distinct population of CNS neurons located predominantly in the raphe nuclei of the brainstem (Dahlstrom and Fuxe, 1964; Steinbusch, 1981; Jacobs and Azmitia, 1992). Although 5-HT neurons are found along the entire length of the raphe nuclei and adjacent reticular formation, from caudal midbrain to caudal medulla, more than half the total population is present in a single midbrain nucleus, the nucleus dorsalis raphe (Wiklund *et al.*, 1981). The dorsal raphe 5-HT neurons, with the substantially smaller population of 5-HT neurons in the adjacent nucleus centralis superior (median raphe), provide the entire 5-HT innervation of forebrain (cf. Jacobs and Azmitia, 1992, for review). The more caudal raphe nuclei project to brainstem, cerebellum and spinal cord. Although there appears to be a limited topography in the dorsal and median raphe projections, individual neurons innervate widespread areas. In this respect, the 5-HT projections of the dorsal and median raphe appear very similar to those of another important monoaminergic cell group innervating the forebrain, the locus coeruleus (Moore and Bloom, 1979). There are unusual aspects, however, of the 5-HT neuron innervation of forebrain. For example, 5-HT neurons of the dorsal raphe provide a dense supraependymal plexus in the third and lateral ventricles (Lorez and Richards, 1973; Aghajamian and Gallagher, 1975) and innervate circumventricular organs such as the organum vasculosum lamina terminalis (Moore, 1977). The innervation of

Obesity Management and Redux^{TM}
ISBN 0-12-518170-1

cerebral cortex is widespread, particularly in superficial layers, with a mean incidence in the rat of one 5-HT terminal to approximately 1000 other cortical terminals (Beaudet and Descarries, 1976). These terminals are unusual in that very few appear to establish conventional synaptic complexes (Descarries *et al.*, 1991), and this is also the case in other forebrain areas such as neostriatum (Soghomonian *et al.*, 1989). Thus, the 5-HT innervation of forebrain is unconventional in several respects.

The function of dorsal raphe neurons appears quite stereotyped and largely associated with changes in behavioural state. Neurons fire regularly and slowly during waking but in drowsiness and slow wave sleep the firing rate decreases and becomes less regular. In rapid eye movement (REM) sleep there is a complete cessation of firing (Jacobs and Azmitia, 1992). Serotonergic neurons are believed to participate in a wide variety of functions (cf. Jacobs and Azmitia, 1992; Jacobs and Fornal, 1995, for reviews). It is of particular interest that the only other activity that is reported to activate some raphe neurons is somatosensory stimulation of the head, face and neck and oral-buccal movements (Fornal *et al.*, 1996).

The function of 5-HT neurons is modified pharmacologically in the therapy of a variety of disorders. Dexfenfluramine therapy for obesity is one such situation. Although there is every indication from extensive postmarketing surveillance and other clinical studies that dexfenfluramine is a safe drug, there have been suggestions from animal studies that there is a potential for neurotoxicity in the use of dexfenfluramine in humans (Ricuarte *et al.*, 1994). In general, these animal studies have used high doses of dexfenfluramine and acute, short-term parenteral administration of the drug. In addition, the major measure of drug effects on 5-HT neurons has been either biochemical assay of brain 5-HT content or immunohistochemistry which cannot distinguish between a neurotoxic effect and the neurochemical depletion of 5-HT from an intact plexus. For these reasons, the present study was undertaken to further clarify this issue. In addition to an immunohistochemical analysis of forebrain 5-HT innervation, the integrity of dorsal raphe neurons was further assessed by counting neuron number and analysing retrograde transport of a standard tracer from the frontal cortex. Retrograde transport is important and useful in this context because the transport of a tracer requires an intact axonal plexus to take up tracer as well as intact transport mechanisms to move the tracer from the terminal plexus to the cell body. Since the 5-HT neurons of the raphe are the only neurons in that region to project to cerebral cortex (Halaris *et al.*, 1976), neurons retrogradely labelled after injection of a tracer into cortex are 5-HT neurons. Thus, retrograde transport is a measure of both the integrity of the forebrain terminal plexus and of an important functional property of the 5-HT neurone, the capacity to transport materials from the axon terminals to the cell body.

METHODS

Adult male albino rats received dexfenfluramine for 21 days by gavage in doses of 2 mg, 4 mg, and 16 mg kg^{-1} day^{-1}. One additional group received gavage administration of vehicle and two groups received vehicle and were pair-fed with the 4 mg and 16 mg kg^{-1} groups, respectively. Four days after completion of the dexfenfluramine administration, bilateral injections of FluoroGold^{TM}, a retrograde tracer, were made into the dorsal frontal cortex at the level of the rostral border of the corpus callosum. Three days thereafter the animals were sacrificed and their brains prepared for immunohistochemical analysis. A second set of animals received FluoroGold injections at 6 months of age and their brains were processed in the same manner as the 7-day animals. Sections through frontal cortex, cingulate cortex, septum, thalamus and hypothalamus, and the midbrain raphe complex, were prepared using an antiserum to serotonin. Sections through the injection site and the midbrain raphe complex were prepared using an antiserum to FluoroGold^{TM}. The density of the 5-HT plexus in dexfenfluramine-treated brains was assessed in comparison with vehicle control and, where appropriate, pair-fed controls by the following criteria. The vehicle control was designated normal innervation. The dexfenfluramine and pair-fed controls were then evaluated with the raters blind to treatment. Each of the forebrain areas noted above was judged as having a 5-HT plexus in one of the following categories: (1) no evident 5-HT fibers; (2) sparse innervation, less than 25% of control; (3) light innervation, 25–50% of control; (4) moderate innervation, 50–75% of control; (5) full innervation, 75–100% of control. 5-Hydroxytryptamine immunoreactive perikarya in the dorsal raphe nucleus were counted using an unbiased stereological method. The results were then converted for each group to per cent of vehicle control. Neurons in the dorsal raphe nucleus retrogradely labelled with FluoroGold were counted and the results also converted to per cent of vehicle control. When the code was broken, all data for the dexfenfluramine-treated animals were compared with those for the pair-fed controls. This is not reported as there is no significant difference from the comparison with the regular vehicle control group.

RESULTS

The results are shown in Table 1 The data for all of the individual forebrain 5-HT plexuses were essentially identical so that these are combined. At 7 days after treatment, there is no difference between vehicle controls and the 2 mg

Table 1

Dexfenfluramine effects on forebrain 5-HT plexuses, raphe 5-HT neuron number and retrograde transport

Treatment group	7-Day survival			6-Month survival		
	Forebrain 5-HT plexus	Raphe 5-HT neuron number	Retro-grade transport	Forebrain 5-HT plexus	Raphe 5-HT neuron number	Retro-grade transport
Vehicle control	100	100	100	100	100	100
2 mg kg^{-1} [a]	98	93	132	97	103	91
4 mg kg^{-1} [a]	97	94	133	100	108	115
16 mg kg^{-1} [a]	50[b]	83	97	85	107	89

[a]Data expressed as per cent vehicle control.
[b]Significantly different from control, $p < 0.02$, Mann-Whitney.

and 4 mg kg^{-1} groups with respect to the density of the 5-HT plexuses. The 16 mg kg^{-1} group shows a significant decrease in density of the plexus with the mean value about 50% of control. However, this decrease in 5-HT plexus density is reversed at 6 months after treatment at which time the density is normal.

There is no alteration of dorsal raphe 5-HT neuron number at any dose level of dexfenfluramine, 2 mg, 4 mg or 16 mg kg^{-1}. Similarly, there is no alteration in retrograde transport. Virtually all of the neurons labelled retrogradely in the midbrain raphe nuclei are in the central region of the dorsal raphe nucleus, and the number of labelled neurons is the same in the 2 mg, 4 mg and 16 mg kg^{-1} dexfenfluramine-treated groups. This demonstrates that the apparent diminution of the plexus in the 16 mg kg^{-1} group does not affect the uptake and transport of a retrograde tracer.

DISCUSSION

Dexfenfluramine has its principal action on 5-HT neurons, producing release of 5-HT and limiting reuptake (Mennini et al., 1991). Administration of dexfenfluramine to animals, even over long periods, can result in a decrease in brain serotonin content that recovers rapidly after cessation of treatment (Duhault and Boulanger, 1977), indicating that the effect may be pharmacological, not neurotoxic. There are instances in animals, however, in which the effects of 5-HT content, particularly with high doses, have been quite prolonged (Kleven and Seiden, 1989; Zaczek et al., 1990; McCann et al.,

1994). These changes have sometimes been interpreted to represent neurotoxicity (cf. McCann *et al.*, 1994, for review). The problem with this interpretation, though, is that it is made by analogy with the effects of other agents, of which 5,7-dihydroxytryptamine is an exemple, which are known to be neurotoxic. The effect common to the two sets of agents, dexfenfluramine on one hand and known 5-HT neuron toxins on the other, is that both can decrease 5-HT content. But, since dexfenfluramine is known to release 5-HT from terminals, a reduction in serotonin content, whether shown neurochemically or immunohistochemically, could represent depletion of transmitter from an intact plexus. This has not yet been resolved. In addition, it was reported some years ego that fenfluramine produces acute morphological changes in raphe 5-HT neurons which were interpreted as neurotoxic (Harvey *et al.*, 1977). No studies have reported a confirmation of this finding but there have been no reported studies which have counted raphe neurons after fenfluramine treatment to show that there is no neuronal loss.

The present study was designed to address these issues. In the first part, the density of the 5-HT plexus was analysed at 7 days and 6 months after dexfenfluramine administration. At doses that approximate 10 times the human therapeutic dose, 2 and 4 mg kg^{-1} day^{-1} to the animals, there are no acute or chronic changes in the forebrain 5-HT plexus. At approximately 30 times the human dose, there is a significant decrease in the 5-HT plexus at 7 days but it is recovered to normal at 6 months. This change with recovery would be in accord with either a drug-induced acute degeneration of the plexus or a depletion of 5-HT from an intact plexus. In order to evaluate this further, the second part of the study was performed. In this, retrograde transport of FluoroGold from the frontal cortex was evaluated in dexfenfluramine-treated and control animals. As noted above, this tests the integrity of the axonal plexus to take up tracer and the functional status of the neuron to transport the tracer to the cell body. No change in retrograde transport was noted either at 7 days or 6 months in any group of the dexfenfluramine-treated animals in comparison with control. The third part of the study examined 5-HT neuron number in the dorsal raphe nucleus. No difference between dexfenfluramine-treated and control animals was observed, indicating that there is no acute or long-term effect of the drug on 5-HT neuron number in the principal nucleus, the dorsal raphe, providing the 5-HT innervation of forebrain.

CONCLUSIONS

Dexfenfluramine has no effect on the 5-HT innervation of the forebrain at doses of 2 and 4 mg kg^{-1} day^{-1} as assessed by morphological methods at 7 days and 6 months after 21 days oral treatment. At 16 mg kg^{-1} day^{-1} there is a significant acute diminution of the density of the forebrain 5-HT plexus which recovers at 6 months. Dexfenfluramine has no effect on 5-HT neuron number in the dorsal raphe nucleus or on the retrograde transport of FluoroGold from the frontal cortex to the dorsal raphe 5-HT neuron perikarya at either 2, 4 or 16 mg kg^{-1} day^{-1} at either 7 days or 6 months after treatment. These data are in accord with the interpretation that dexfenfluramine in doses in the range of 10 times the human therapeutic dose has no acute or chronic effect on the morphological integrity of 5-HT neurons innervating forebrain. At doses approximating 30 times the human dose, there is an acute decrease in the density of the forebrain 5-HT innervation without an effect on retrograde transport or dorsal raphe 5-HT neuron number. This recovers by 6 months, suggesting that the acute effect on the plexus reflects depletion of 5-HT from an otherwise intact plexus.

REFERENCES

Aghajanian GK, Gallagher DW (1975) Raphe origin of serotonergic nerves terminating in the cerebral ventricles. *Brain Res* **88**: 221–231.

Beaudet A, Descarries L (1976) Quantitative data on serotonin nerve terminals in adult rat cortex. *Brain Res* **111**: 301–309.

Dahlstrom A, Fuxe K (1964) Evidence for the existence of monoamine neurons in the central nervous system. I. Demonstration of monoamines in the cell bodies of brain stem neurons. *Acta Physiol Scand* **62** (suppl. 232): 1–55.

Descarries L, Seguela P, Watkins KC (1991) Nonjunctional relationships of monoamine axon terminals in the cerebral cortex of the adult rat. In: Fuxe K and Agnati LF (eds) *Volume Transmission in the Brain*. Raven Press, New York: 53–62.

Duhault J, Boulanger M (1977) Fenfluramine long-term administration and brain serotonin. *Eur J Pharmacol* **43**: 203–205.

Fornal LA, Metzler CW, Marrosu F, Ribiero-do-Valle LE, Jacobs BL (1996) A subgroup of dorsal raphe serotonergic neurons in the cat is strongly activated during oral-buccal movements. *Brain Res* **716**: 123–133.

Halaris AE, Jones BE, Moore RY (1976) Axonal transport in serotonin neurons of the midbrain raphe. *Brain Res* **107**: 555–574.

Harvey JA, McMaster SE, Fuller RW (1977) Comparison between the neurotoxic and serotonin-depleting effects of various halogenated derivatives of amphetamines in the rat. *J Pharmacol Exp Ther* **202**: 581–589.

Jacobs BL, Azmitia EL (1992) Structure and function of the brain serotonin system. *Physiol Rev* **72**: 165–229.

Jacobs BL, Fornal C (1995) Serotonin and behavior: A general hypothesis. In: Bloom FE and Kupfer DJ (eds), *Psychopharmacology: The Fourth Generation of Progress*. Raven Press, New York: 461–469.

Kleven MS, Seiden LS (1989) D-, L- and DL-fenfluramine cause long-lasting depletions of serotonin in rat brain. *Brain Res* **505**: 351–359.

Lorez HP, Richards JG (1973) Distribution of indolealkylamine nerve terminals in ventricles of the rat brain. *Z Zellforsch* **144**: 511–522

McCann U, Hatzidimitriou G, Ridenour A *et al.* (1994) Dexfenfluramine and serotonin neurotoxicity: Further pre-clinical evidence that clinical caution is indicated. *J Pharmacol Exp Ther* **269**: 792–798.

Mennini T, Bizzi A, Caccia S *et al.* (1991) Comparative studies on the anorectic activity of d-fenfluramine in mice, rats and guinea pigs. *Naunyn–Schmiedeberg's Arch. Pharmacol* **343**: 485–490

Moore RY (1977) Organum vasculosum lamina terminalis: Innervation by serotonin neurons of the midbrain raphe. *Neurosci Lett* **5**: 297–302.

Moore RY, Bloom FE (1979) Central catecholamine neuron systems: Anatomy and physiology of the norepinephrine and epinephrine systems. *Ann Rev Neurosci* **2**: 113–168.

Soghomonian JJ, Descarries L, Watkins KC (1989) Serotonin innervation in adult rat neostriatum. II. Ultrastructural features: A radioautographic and immunocyto-chemical study. *Brain Res* **481**: 67–86.

Steinbusch HWM (1981) Distribution of serotonin-immunoreactivity in the central nervous system of the rat cell bodies and terminals. *Neurosci* **6**: 557–618.

Wiklund L, Leger L, Persson M (1981) Monoamine cell distribution in the cat brain. *J Comp Neurol* **203**: 613–647.

Zaczek R, Battaglia G, Culp S, Appel NM, Contrera JF, DeSouza, EB (1990) Effects of repeated fenfluramine administration on indexes of monoamine function in rat brain: Pharmacokinetic, dose response, regional specificity and time course data. *J Pharmacol Exp Ther* **253**: 104–112.

Behavioural and Other Functional Effects of Low and High Doses of Fenfluramine and Dexfenfluramine

Stanley A. Lorens

Professor of Pharmacology and Neuroscience, Department of Pharmacology and Experimental Therapeutics, Loyola University Chicago Medical Center, 2160 South First Avenue, Maywood, IL 60153, USA

INTRODUCTION

Fenfluramine and dexfenfluramine are used clinically worldwide as anorectic agents. This contribution summarizes studies, primarily originating in the author's laboratory, which have addressed potential functional and behavioural side and potentially toxic effects of fenfluramine and dexfenfluramine. These can be identified and discussed under two rubrics:

(1) effects associated with therapeutic doses;
(2) effects which are a consequence of overdosage.

Review of the available preclinical and clinical literature leads one to the following conclusions.

(1) Administration of either low or high doses of fenfluramine and dexfenfluramine does *not* produce any significant or consistent adverse functional or behavioural effects.
(2) Fenfluramine and dexfenfluramine do *not* produce neurotoxic effects according to functional/behavioural criteria (see Abou-Donia, 1992; Tilson and Harry, 1992).

Obesity Management and Redux[TM]
ISBN 0-12-518170-1

FUNCTIONAL EFFECTS OF LOW DOSES

Learning and memory

We (Lorens *et al.*, 1991) have shown that daily administration of low doses of dexfenfluramine (beginning 30 days prior to testing, throughout behavioural testing, and until sacrifice 11 weeks later) to young (5–7 months of age; 1.2 mg kg^{-1} day^{-1}, p.o., in the animals' drinking water) and old (19–21 months of age; 0.6 mg kg^{-1} day^{-1}, p.o.) male Fisher 344 (F344) rats does not affect the acquisition of a one-way (place) conditioned avoidance response (CAR) or the acquisition of a two-way visually discriminated CAR. These data suggest that subchronic low dose of dexfenfluramine would not affect learning processes in either young or elderly patients.

Immunological competence

Subchronic administration (30–38 days) of dexfenfluramine (0.6–1.8 mg kg^{-1} day^{-1}, p.o.) to young (5 months) and old (21 months) male and female F344 rats has been shown to dose-dependently augment T and B lymphocyte functions, to increase cell-mediated cytotoxicity for natural killer cell (NK) tumour targets, and to enhance cell-mediated activities for opportunistic microbial pathogens in an age- and sex-dependent manner (Clancy *et al.*, 1991; Petrovic *et al.*, 1991; Lorens *et al.*, 1993c; Clancy and Lorens, 1996; Mathews *et al.*, 1996). Further, chronic exposure (8 months) of ageing male F344 rats to dexfenfluramine (0.6 mg kg^{-1} day^{-1}, p.o. beginning at the age of 15 months) enabled their NK and T cell responsiveness to remain at young 7 month control levels. This observation was of particular interest since the old dexfenfluramine-treated animals showed a significant decrease in pathology, especially in the spleen (Clancy and Lorens, 1996).

The augmentation of NK activity and the increase in lymphocyte proliferation produced by dexfenfluramine (Clancy *et al.*, 1991; Petrovic *et al.*, 1991; Lorens *et al.*, 1993c; Clancy and Lorens, 1996) presumably is due to increased availability of serotonin (5-HT) at receptors located in the immune and/or the nervous system (Clancy *et al.*, 1993; Lorens *et al.*, 1993a,c). Dexfenfluramine also appears to increase the influx of lymphocytes into lymph nodes and to enhance the overall antifungal activity of lymphocytes at the site of infection (Mathews *et al.*, 1996). *In vivo,* dexfenfluramine appears to bias the protective immune response toward the T cell compartment of the immune system during localized *Candida albicans* infection. *In vivo,* 5-HT has been reported to stimulate NK activity in human percoll-fractionated peripheral blood lymphocytes (Hellstrand and Hermodsson, 1990). B and T lymphocyte functions as measured by lymphoproliferation have been shown to correlate with augmentation of the adaptive immune system. Cell-mediated cytotoxicity for NK targets and for opportunistic microbial pathogens are thought to be a consequence of the innate immune system. These observations suggest that low therapeutic doses of dexfenfluramine will not impair immune functions in humans.

Stress and plasma hormone levels

It is well known that the acute administration of fenfluramine and dexfenflur-amine can cause the release of several hypophysial releasing factors and trophic hormones as well as stimulate renin secretion (Van de Kar *et al.*, 1985a,b; Van de Kar, 1991). In addition, repeated daily administration leads to the rapid development of tolerance to the endocrinological effects of dexfenfluramine (see, e.g. Serri and Rasio, 1989; Handa *et al.*, 1993). We have found, moreover, that subchronic treatment with low doses of dexfenfluramine (0.2–0.6 mg kg^{-1} day^{-1}, p.o., in the animals' drinking water) does not adversely affect basal hormone (prolactin, ACTH and corticosterone) levels in either young or old F344 rats of both sexes. In fact, subchronic dexfenfluramine treatment normalizes the exaggerated ACTH/corticosterone response to novelty stress in old male animals and attenuates the enhanced prolactin response to stress in old female rats (Handa *et al.*, 1993, 1994). Extrapolation of these animal data to humans suggests that patients receiving low therapeutic doses of dexfenfluramine should not experience any significant endocrinologi-cal side effects.

COMPARISON OF THE BEHAVIOURAL EFFECTS OF 5,7-DHT AND HIGH DOSES OF FENFLURAMINE

Our laboratory (supported by funds obtained from the National Institute of Drug Abuse) has shown that the administration of repeated high doses of fenfluramine (5–20 mg kg^{-1}, s.c., b.i.d. × 4 days) to young (4–7 months of age at sacrifice) Sprague–Dawley and/or F344 male rats does not lead to behavioural dysfunctions when measured 2–10 weeks post injection. Thus, fenfluramine does not affect:

(1) exploratory behaviour (20 min exposure to a novel open field/holeboard) (Hata *et al.*, 1989; Lorens *et al.*, 1990a,b; Hata and Lorens, 1996);

(2) motor coordination or stamina (12 min swim test) (Hata *et al.*, 1989; Lorens *et al.*, 1990a,b, 1993b);
(3) defensive behaviour towards an intruder into the home cage (territorial defence) (Lorens *et al.*, 1993b);
(4) the acquisition of a one-way (place) or visually discriminated two-way (non-spatial, shuttlebox) conditioned avoidance response (CAR) (Lorens *et al.*, 1993b);
(5) spatial memory formation and its extinction in an eight-arm radial maze (Lorens *et al.*, 1990a, 1993b; Hata and Lorens, 1996); or
(6) thermal (50°C hot plate) pain sensitivity and morphine (5.0 mg kg^{-1}, s.c.; hot plate test) analgesia (Hata *et al.*, 1989; Hata and Lorens 1996).

These observations indicate that fenfluramine does not produce functional or behavioural neurotoxicity according to accepted criteria (see Abou-Donia, 1992; Tilson and Harry, 1992). Furthermore, the classical serotonin neurotoxin, 5,7-dihydroxytryptamine (5,7-DHT), unlike dexfenfluramine or fenfluramine:

(1) produces hyperaggressivity as measured by increased home cage offensive (territorial defence) behaviour toward an intruder rat (Vergnes *et al.*, 1988; Lorens *et al.*, 1993b);
(2) enhances morphine analgesia (Hata *et al.*, 1989; Hata and Lorens, 1996); and,
(3) can impair swimming ability as well as reduce exploratory behaviour (Mackenzie *et al.*, 1978; Gately *et al.*, 1985, 1986; Lorens *et al.*, 1989, 1990a,b, 1993c).

5,7-DHT also enhances the behavioural responses (forepaw treading, flat body posture, head twitches and defaecation) produced by injection of the 5-HT precursor, 5-hydroxytryptophan (5-HTP). High doses of dexfenfluramine and fenfluramine have no effect on these 5-HTP-induced stereotypic behaviours (Lategan *et al.*, 1989). These results confirm the reported supersensitive behavioural response to 5-HTP 2–4 weeks following administration of 5,7-DHT, but not after fenfluramine treatment (Clineschmidt *et al.*, 1978).

ABUSE LIABILITY

It is *very important* to note that fenfluramine and dexfenfluramine, in stark contrast to *d*- and methamphetamine, as well as cocaine, do *not* serve as a positive reinforcer in animal and human drug self-administration paradigms

(Götestam and Gunne, 1972; Woods and Tessel, 1974; Griffiths *et al.*, 1978a,b; Johanson and Uhlenhuth, 1982; Papasava *et al.*, 1986). Administration of high doses of fenfluramine and dexfenfluramine to humans, furthermore, induces dysphoria (Griffith *et al.*, 1976). Thus, fenfluramine and dexfenfluramine do not exhibit abuse potential, making euphoria-motivated self-induced overdosage most unlikely. Based on these preclinical and human studies the FDA Drug Abuse Advisory Committee recommended (29 September 1995) that fenfluramine and its isomers be descheduled.

CONCLUSIONS

The literature reviewed above, coupled with the data obtained via Phase IV surveillance, leads to the conclusion that fenfluramine and dexfenfluramine are virtually devoid of any significant side or toxic effects (Lorens *et al.*, 1994). In short, there is no evidence extant that fenfluramine and dexfenfluramine produce functional toxicity.

REFERENCES

Abou-Donia MB (1992) Principles and methods for evaluating neurotoxicity. In: Abou-Donia MB (ed.) *Neurotoxicology*. CRC Press, Boca Raton, Florida 509–525.

Clancy J Jr, Lorens SA (1996) Subchronic and chronic exposure to d-fenfluramine dose-dependently enhances splenic immune functions in young and old male Fischer-344 rats. *Behav Brain Res* 73: 355–358.

Clancy J Jr, Petrovic LM, Gordon BH, Handa RJ, Campbell DB, Lorens SA (1991) Effects of subchronic dexfenfluramine on splenic immune functions in young and old male and female Fischer 344 rats. *Int J Immunopharmacol* 13: 1203–1212.

Clancy J Jr, Fillion G, Hellstrand K, Lorens SA (1993) Interactions between serotonin and the immune system: An overview. In: Paoletti R, Vanhoutte P, Saxena P (eds) *Serotonin from Cell Biology to Pharmacology and Therapeutics II*. Kluwer Academics Publishers, Dordrecht: 353–357.

Clineschmidt BV, Zacchei AG, Totaro JA, Pflueger AB, McGuffin JC, Wishousky TI (1978) Fenfluramine and brain serotonin. *Ann NY Acad Sci* 305: 222–241.

Gately PF, Poon SL, Segal DS, Geyer MA (1985) Depletion of brain serotonin by 5,7-dihydroxytryptamine alters the response to amphetamine and the habituation of locomotor activity in rats. *Psychopharmacology* 87: 400–405.

Gately PF, Segal DS, Geyer MA (1986) The behavioural effects of depletions of brain serotonin induced by 5,7-dihydroxytryptamine vary with time after administration. *Behav Neural Biol* 45: 31–42.

Götestam KG, Gunne L-M (1972) Subjective effects of two anorexigenic agents fenfluramine and AN 448 in amphetamine-dependent subjects. *Br J Addict* 67: 39–44.

Griffith JD, Nutt JG, Jasinski DR (1976) A comparison of fenfluramine and amphetamine in man. *Clin Pharmacol Ther* **18**: 563–570.

Griffiths RR, Brady JV, Snell JD (1978a) Progressive-ratio performance maintained by drug infusions: Comparison of cocaine, diethylpropion, chlorphentermine, and fenfluramine. *Psychopharmacology* **56**: 5–13.

Griffiths RR, Brady JV, Snell JD (1978b) Relationship between anorectic and reinforcing properties of appetite suppressant drugs: Implications for assessment of abuse liability. *Biol Psychiat* **13**: 283–290.

Handa RJ, Cross MK, George M *et al.* (1993) Neuroendocrine and neurochemical responses to novelty stress in young and old male F344 rats: Effects of dexfenfluramine treatment. *Pharmacol Biochem Behav* **46**: 101–109.

Handa RJ, Cross MK, George M *et al.* (1994) Neuroendocrine and neurochemical responses to novelty stress in young and old female F344 rats: Effects of dexfenfluramine treatment. *Physiol Behav* **55**: 117–124.

Hata N, Lorens SA (1996) Behavioral and neurochemical effects of 5,7-dihydroxytryptamine (5,7-DHT), (±)3,4-methylenedioxymethamphetamine (MDMA) and (±)fenfluramine in male rats. *Psychopharmacology* (in prep.).

Hata N, Cabrera T, Lorens S (1989) A comparison of the behavioural and neurochemical effects of 5,7-DHT, MDMA and d,l-fenfluramine. *Neurosci Abstr* **15**: 1186.

Hellstrand K, Hermodsson S (1990) Enhancement of human natural killer cell cytotoxicity by serotonin: Role of non-T/CD16[+] NK cells, accessory monocytes, and 5-HT$_{1A}$ receptors. *Cell Immunol* **127**: 199–209.

Johanson CE, Uhlenhuth CE (1982) Drug preferences in humans. *Fed Proc* **41**: 228–233.

Lategan A, Koek WW, Bervoets K, Jackson A, Lehmann J, Colpaert FC (1989) Differential effects of fenfluramine and 5,7-dihydroxytryptamine on the 1-5-hydroxytryptophan-induced serotonin syndrome in rats. Presented at the International Symposium on Serotonin from Cell Biology to Pharmacology and Therapeutics, Abstract Book, p. 36.

Lorens SA, Hata N, Cabrera T, Hamilton ME (1989) Behavioral effects of 5,7-DHT and MDMA in rats. In: Paoletti R, Vanhoutte P, Brunello N and Maggi F (eds) *Serotonin from Cell Biology to Pharmacology and Therapeutics*. Kluwer Academic Publishers, The Netherlands: pp. 615–623.

Lorens SA, Hata N, Cabrera T, Hamilton ME (1990a) Comparison of the behavioural and neurochemical effects of 5,7-DHT, MDMA and d,l-fenfluramine. Proceedings of the 51st Annual Scientific meeting, Committee on Problems of Drug Dependence, Inc. *NIDA Research Monograph: Problems of Drug Dependence 1989* **95**: 347.

Lorens SA, Hata N, Handa RJ, Cabrera T (1990b) Functional consequences of selective CNS serotonin depletion: A comparison of methods. *Psychopharmacology* **101** (suppl.): S34).

Lorens SA, George M, Hejna G (1991) Subchronic dexfenfluramine treatment does not affect avoidance conditioning in young and old Fischer 344 male rats. Research report submitted to IRIS, France.

Lorens SA, George M, Dersch C, Clancy J, Zaczek R (1993a) Age- and sex-dependent effects of (+)fenfluramine (dexfenfluramine) on splenic monoamine metabolism, receptors and immune function. *Neurosci Abstr* **19**: 949.

Lorens SA, Hata N, George M, Hejna G (1993b) Functional and neurochemical correlates of the substituted amphetamines: A comparison with 6-hydroxydopamine (6-OHDA) and 5,7-dihydroxytryptamine (5,7-DHT). Presented at the ICN Sponsored Satellite Meeting on *Cellular and Molecular*

Mechanisms of Drug Abuse: Cocaine and Methamphetamine (Nice, France) August.

Lorens SA, Petrovic L, Hejna G, Dong XW, Clancy J Jr (1993c) The stimulatory effects of a dexfenfluramine (dexfenfluramine) on blood and splenic immune functions in the Fischer 344 rat are age and sex dependent. In: Paoletti R, Vanhoutte P and Saxena P (eds) *Serotonin from Cell Biology to Pharmacology and Therapeutics II*. Kluwer Academic Publishers: The Netherlands: 337–343.

Lorens SA, Hata N, George M, Hejna G (1994) Are the substituted amphetamines neurotoxic? Comparison with 6-hydroxydopamine (6-OHDA), and 5,7-dihydroxytryptamine (5,7-DHT). *NeuroToxicology* **15**: 213.

Mackenzie RG, Hoebel BG, Norelli C, Trulson ME (1978) Increased tilt-cage activity after serotonin depletion by 5,7-dihydroxytryptamine. *Neuropharmacology* **17**: 957–963.

Mathews HL, Lorens SA, Clancy J Jr (1996) Effect of d-fenfluramine on the local immune response to the opportunistic microbial pathogen *Candida albicans*. *Behav Brain Res* **73**: 369–374.

Papasava M, Singer G, Papasava C (1986) Food deprivation fails to potentiate intravenous self-administration of fenfluramine in naive rats. *Appetite* **7**: 55–61.

Petrovic LM, Lorens SA, George M, Cabrera T, Gordon B, Handa RJ, Campbell B, Clancey J Jr (1991) Subchronic dexfenfluramine treatment enhances the immunological competence of old female Fischer 344 rats. In: Fozard JR and Saxena PR (eds) *Serotonin: Molecular Biology, Receptors and Functional Effects*. Birkhauser-Verlag, Basel: 389–397.

Serri O. Rasio E (1989) Temporal changes in prolactin and corticosterone response during chronic treatment with dexfenfluramine. *Hormone Res* **31**: 180–183.

Tilson HA, Harry GJ (1992) Neurobehavioural toxicology. In: Abou-Donia MB (ed) *Neurotoxicology*. CRC Press, Boca Raton, Florida: 527–571.

Van de Kar LD (1991) Neuroendocrine pharmacology of serotonergic (5-HT) neurons. *Ann Rev Pharmacol Toxicol* **31**: 289–420.

Van de Kar LD, Richardson KD, Urban JH (1985a) Serotonin and norepinephrine-dependent effects of fenfluramine on plasma renin activity in conscious male rats. *Neuropharmacology* **24**: 487–494.

Van de Kar LD, Urban JH, Richardson KD, Bethea CL (1985b) Pharmacological studies on the serotoninergic and nonserotonin-mediated stimulation of prolactin and corticosterone secretion by fenfluramine. *Neuroendocrinology* **41**: 283–288.

Vergnes M, Depaulis A, Boehrer A, Kempf E (1988) Selective increase in offensive behavior in the rat following intrahypothalamic 5,7-DHT-induced serotonin depletion. *Behav Brain Res* **29**: 85–91.

Woods JH, Tessel RE (1974) Fenfluramine: amphetamine congener that fails to maintain drug-taking behavior in the rhesus monkey. *Science* **185**: 1067–1069 .

The Use of Pharmacokinetics in the Assessment of Dexfenfluramine Safety

B. Campbell

Servier Research and Development, Fulmer Hall, Windmill Road, Fulmer, Slough SL3 6HH, UK

B. Dard-Brunelle

Institut de Recherches Internationales Servier, 6 place des Pléiades, 92415 Courbevoie Cedex, France

S. Caccia

Istituto di Ricerche Farmacologiche Mario Negri, Via Eritrea 62, 20157 Milan, Italy

All animals are not equal and some are less equal than others
(apologies to George Orwell)

INTRODUCTION

For many years, it has been well documented that high doses of fenfluramine, and more recently dexfenfluramine, reduce the levels of serotonin (5-HT) and its metabolite 5-hydroxy indole acetic acid (5-HIAA) in the brain of animals (Clineschmidt *et al.*, 1978; Invernizzi *et al.*, 1986; Kleven *et al.*, 1988). This effect may be transient at low doses in rats (<4 mg kg^{-1}) or continue for months at high doses (48 mg kg^{-1}) (Zaczek et al., 1990) and the duration is probably dependent on the initial fall (Fracasso et al., 1995). It had been thought that this reduction in brain 5-HT was necessary for the drug to reduce food intake by a combination of competitive inhibition of 5-HT uptake and release (Fuller et al., 1988), but evidence has shown that brain indole concentrations are either not changed in mice (Carlton and Rowland, 1989) or may be increased in rat whole brain (Zaczek et al., 1990) or synapse (Schwartz et al., 1989) at pharmacological doses ($\sim$2–6 mg kg^{-1}) which reduce food intake (Hoebel et al., 1991). Thus, the doses employed to affect these neurotransmitters so dramatically can be thought of as being overdosage. It is interesting that this effect is not peculiar to dexfenfluramine and is seen with many compounds which alter 5-HT metabolism, including other substituted phenylethylamines and fluoxetine, if the doses are raised sufficiently high and the animals do not die (Trouvin et al., 1993).

These reductions in central 5-HT levels, particularly in the cortex, which appears to be more sensitive compared with other brain regions, have led some investigators to suggest that the drug is neurotoxic (Kleven et al., 1988; McCann et al., 1995). This hypothesis has been put forward because immuno-fluorescent examination of cortical sections stained for the presence of 5-HT found a significant reduction in the number of serotoninergic neurons and some that appeared swollen (Molliver and Molliver, 1990). These observations were not surprising since this is an indirect immunofluorescence method and without the presence of 5-HT within the neuron, the neuron itself could not be visualized and, below a certain threshold concentration, fully intact axons cannot be seen (S. Lorens, pers. comm.). In any case, other workers have shown that these swellings return to normal after 15–30 days (Sotelo, 1991) even at high doses (16 mg kg^{-1}) (Kalia, 1991, 1992), confirming the continued presence of the neuron. Uptake sites are also reduced, but this is not necessarily related to the reduction in 5-HT (Zaczek et al., 1990) and it has been argued (Baumgarten et al., 1992) that this could be explained by a downregulation of these receptors. Other workers have searched for more functional indices of neuronal damage, including cell body loss by Nissl staining (Oliver et al., 1978; Sotelo and Zamora, 1979) or counting neurons in the raphe (Rattray et al., 1994; Moore, this volume), reduced retrograde transport (Kalia and O'Malley, 1993; Kalia, 1996), glial activation by measurement of GFAP (O'Callaghan and Miller, 1994; O'Callaghan, 1996), neuronal regeneration as measured by GAP 43 (Rose et al., 1996), persistent reduction in mRNA of tryptophan hydroxylase (Bendotti et al., 1993) and persistent behavioural modification (Lorens et al., 1993; Raleigh et al., 1986), but none have been able to show effects which are indicative of neuro-degeneration.

Other compounds, such as methylenedioxymethamphetamine (MDMA), p-chloroamphetamine   (PCA)   or   the   known   neurotoxin,   5,7-

dihydroxytriptamine (5,7-DHT), can reduce 5-HT but also cause some degree of measurable neurotoxicity and the difference between the effects of these compounds and that of fenfluramine is that whilst these modify dopamine turnover (Schmidt, 1992), the effect of fenfluramine is primarily serotonergic.

THE PROBLEM

The long-term 5-HT/5-HIAA reductions with fenfluramine at high doses, however, cannot be readily explained and, when comparing these effects in different species in terms of dosage, the primate appears to be more sensitive compared with the rat, whilst the mouse is the least sensitive. Thus, there has been concern that, in humans, there may similarly be a long-term reduction in 5-HT when the drug is administered therapeutically (McCann *et al.*, 1994), even though no behavioural changes associated with such a reduction has been reported, despite usage in millions of patients for more than 30 years.

Such extrapolation of effects from the animal experimental results to those that might occur in humans must rely on at least two basic assumptions: (1) there are no species differences in the mechanism of action and sensitivity of the response and (2) there are no species differences in the pharmacokinetics and metabolism and that the same dose gives the same brain levels of active compounds.

SPECIES DIFFERENCES IN BIODISPOSITION

It is well documented for many drugs that there are major species differences in the kinetics and clearance from the body in terms of both rate and route. Indeed, from allometric or body size considerations, it can be expected that small animals will remove drugs more rapidly from the body because of their relatively faster tissue blood flows and larger organs when expressed as a percentage of body size (Boxembaum, 1982). For renal excretion, these differences are proportional to body surface area or overall metabolic rate, whilst for those drugs which are predominately metabolized with a slow clearance, elimination is more proportional to a function of body weight and maximum life potential (Campbell, 1995). In general, smaller animals eliminate drugs more rapidly, but for those that are metabolized more extensively, active/toxic metabolites are subsequently produced. In addition, different species have now been shown to have different phase I cytochrome P450 oxidative metabolic enzymes and often the metabolic routes and corresponding metabolites can show large interspecies variability. The interpretation of this data becomes even more confusing when the metabolites produced are not only active but elicit their effect through different mechanisms. Thus, the common method of extrapolating a dosage that exhibits an effect in animals to the dosage used in humans, and expecting the same effect to occur without at least blood or tissue levels of the active components, is often a misrepresentation of the data. Dexfenfluramine is no exception.

METABOLISM

The plasma pharmacokinetics and metabolism of dexfenfluramine has been studied in at least eight species, including human. In general, the peak levels are comparable but because the half-life is related to a function of body weight, the clearance is faster in the smaller rodents compared to the larger primates (Fig. 1).

The metabolism of fenfluramine has been extensively studied using both radioactive (^{14}C) (Marchant et al., 1992) and cold gas liquid chromatography (GLC) (Caccia et al., 1982) analytical techniques and it has shown that the only major circulating active metabolite of fenfluramine is the dealkyl derivative, norfenfluramine. The measurement of this compound is important since it is thought to have a greater contributory role to 5-HT depletion compared with that of the parent drug (Johnson and Nichols, 1990; Caccia et al., 1993) because of a more prominent activity on release of vesicular stored 5-HT (Mennini et al., 1991). The extent of this active metabolite formation can be measured by comparing the ratios of the areas under the plasma time curves for dexnorfenfluramine and dexfenfluramine (Campbell, 1991). This metabolic ratio shows marked interspecies differences (Fig. 2) and is less than 1 for mice and men, with a predominance of the parent drug, and as high as 25–30 for some non-human primates, indicating a predominance of the metabolite. These metabolic ratios are calculated after a single dose, but the normal regimen to maximize the 5-HT depletion is to administer the drug twice daily for 4 days and, under these conditions, the species differences in metabolism are even more exaggerated.

LINEAR KINETICS

In the extrapolation of high dose data from animals to humans, it is also assumed that the blood or tissue levels will increase proportionally to the dose and that the kinetics are therefore linear. Increasingly, we are becoming aware that this may be the exception rather than the rule and that due to non-linear saturation in clearance, higher doses lead to disproportionately higher drug levels. This is the case with fenfluramine in rats; an increase of 24 times in the dose produces a 120 times increase in plasma, and correspondingly, in brain levels (Fig. 3). Similar non-linearity can be expected in other species over a wide dosage range, whilst in humans the dose is fixed (30 mg day^{-1}) and this does not become a problem.

BRAIN UPTAKE

Rarely is it possible to measure the drug levels in the tissue of activity but, since brain levels of 5-HT have been routinely measured in these animal experiments, it has been comparatively easy to measure at the same time the uptake of dexfenfluramine and dexnorfenfluramine into the brain. It is usually assumed that the brain uptake for drugs is similar across the species, but once more we find that this is not the case for dexfenfluramine. It appears to be again related to the species body weight. Thus, the rodents have a high brain-to-plasma ratio of 30–60, whilst for the monkeys it is 15–20, and for humans it was less than 10. The animal data came from controlled studies where the administered doses were known. This was not possible in humans since the original data came from two individuals who had committed suicide by taking large fenfluramine overdoses (>40 mg kg^{-1}) (Fleisher and Campbell, 1969; Holmes and Gordon, 1989).

Clearly, because of the importance of this preliminary finding, it was necessary to confirm these data in more subjects and at therapeutic doses. The problem was how to measure the levels inside the brains of living subjects. Dexfenfluramine has a trifluoromethyl substitution on the phenyl ring and tissue fluorine atoms (^{18}F) can be measured externally by nuclear magnetic resonance spectroscopy or imaging (MRS or MRI) without the need to administer radioactive material, as would have been the case with positron emission tomography (PET). This method has been used previously to measure the brain levels of different antidepressants, such as fluoxetine (Renshaw et al., 1992) and trifluoperazine (Karson et al., 1992), which also contain fluorine.

Eleven obese subjects were administered dexfenfluramine (30 mg day^{-1}: ~0.3 mg kg^{-1}) for 3 months and the brain levels of both dexfenfluramine and dexnorfenfluramine were measured together since it was not possible to separate their individual signals. There was little inter- or intra-subject variability in brain concentrations and, from Fig. 4, it can be seen that after 10 days, steady-state levels had been reached in both the brain and plasma (measured by GLC), remaining constant for 3 months (mean peak brain levels

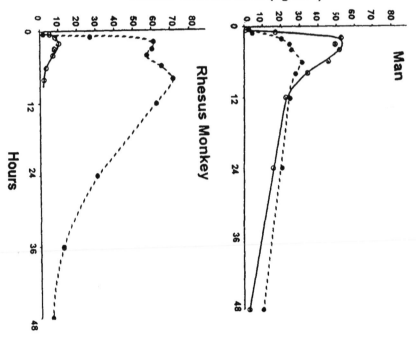

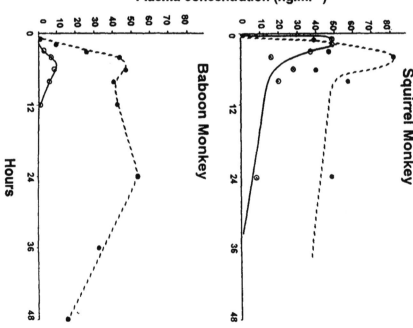

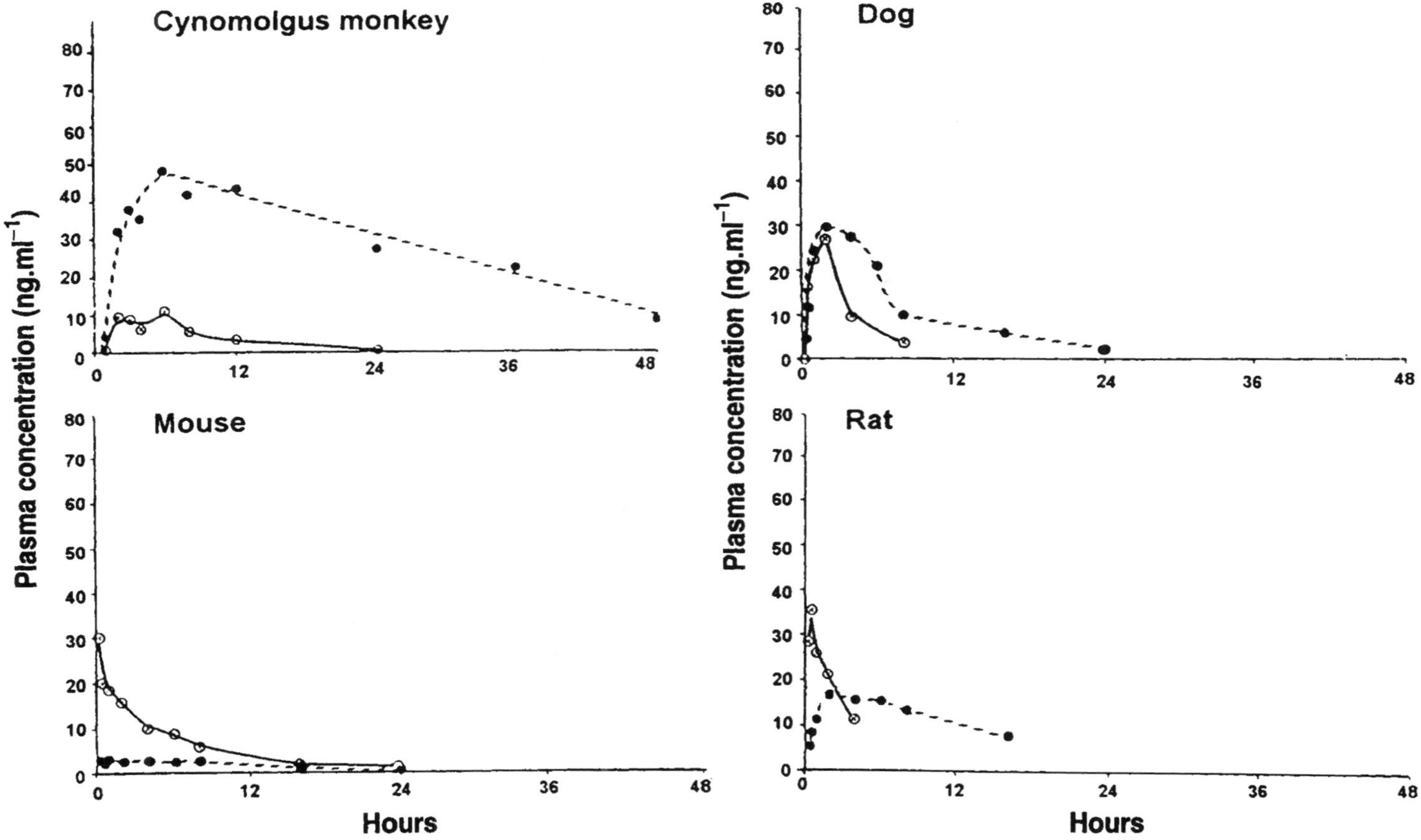

Fig. 1   Interspecies comparison in the plasma kinetics of dexfenfluramine (○——○) and dexnorfenfluramine (●----●) (data normalized to 1 mg kg^{-1})

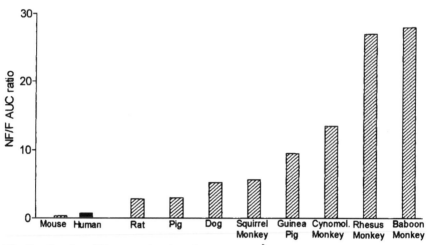

Fig 2. Species differences in the plasma area under the curve metabolic ratio (dexnorfenfluramine/dexfenfluramine) following single oral doses (guinea pig i.p.).

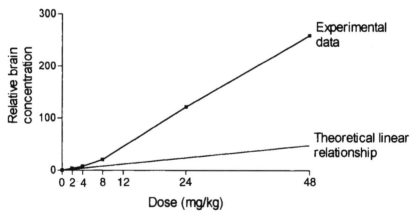

Fig. 3. Comparison of the expected linear proportional relationship between dose and brain concentration and experimental data in rats administered different doses of fenfluramine (subcutaneous) b.i.d. for 4 days.

4.2 ± 0.2 μM; plasma levels 0.25 ± 0.07 μM), indicating no long-term accumulation (Christensen *et al.*, 1995). Rarely can these methods be standardized and normally it is assumed that the resonance signal inside the skull is unaffected by bone or cerebral tissue. In this study, the measurements were standardized by administering dexfenfluramine to three rhesus monkeys for

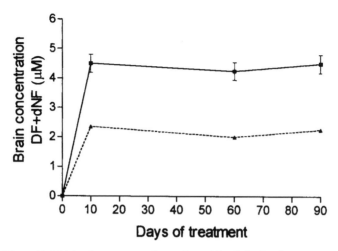

Fig. 4.   Mean (±SD) brain concentrations of combined dexfenfluramine + dexnorfenfluramine in obese patients measured by MRS following daily administration of 30 mg dexfenfluramine (▲-----▲ corrected values).

4 days to reach equilibrium, and the brain levels measured by MRS were compared with the absolute levels obtained by excision of brain tissue and analysis by the specific GLC procedure. However, when corrections were made for the muscle, blood vessels, etc. that which are counted in addition to the skull in the smaller primate brain, it was found that although the MRS gave a reasonable estimate of the brain levels, it did tend to overestimate the concentrations by approximately 50%. The corrected mean human brain levels of combined dexfenfluramine and dexnorfenfluramine from the 11 subjects over the 90 days of treatment would now be 2.2 μM. Interestingly, the brain-to-plasma ratio calculated using this figure (B/P = 8) agrees very closely with that obtained from the overdose cases (B/P = 9), providing further validation that brain levels obtained by this method are acceptable and that the brain uptake may be constant over a wide dosage range, at least in humans.

Thus a good estimate of the brain levels in humans at steady-state levels had been obtained in 11 subjects, but it was not certain that this minimal intersubject variability would be found in a larger population of patients. As part of the Index study (International trial of long-term dexfenfluramine in obesity: Guy-Grand *et al.*, 1989), a double-blind 12 month placebo-controlled European clinical trial involving more than 800 patients, plasmas were taken at 6 and 12 month intervals to measure drug levels. At 6 months, in 339 treated patients who provided samples, the mean ± SEM for dexfenfluramine was 21.0 ± 0.9 ng ml^{-1} and for dexnorfenfluramine was 13.1 ± 0.6 ng ml^{-1}, whilst at 12 months, in 264 patients, the values were respectively 19.2 ± 1.0 ng ml^{-1} and 11.3 ± 0.6 ng ml^{-1}. The combined mean of the sum of dexfenfluramine and dexnorfenfluramine became 0.15 when expressed as μM. This is less than that found in the magnetic resonance spectroscopy (MRS) study, possibly due to the lack of compliance (as many as 25% of subjects had values less than 6 ng ml^{-1} for both compounds). The range of combined levels in the Index study was 0–156 ng ml^{-1}, equivalent to 0.6 μM, but such high values (>100 ng ml^{-1}) were observed in only five subjects. When the analysis was repeated on a second occasion, only one subject had again high values, suggesting that the results for the others could be artifactual.

SPECIES DIFFERENCES IN ACTIVITY

As discussed previously, dexfenfluramine has little direct effect on the indices of neuronal function and that the main concern is the possibility of long-term 5-HT/5-HIAA reduction. With good approximations of the actual drug levels in human brain after therapeutic doses, it should now be possible to determine indirectly if these levels could lower these indoles. But which species should be used as a comparison, since previous workers have suggested that there are important species differences in sensitivity? When all the data from primates and rodents are put together and the relationship between brain levels and the changes in 5-HT compared (Fig. 5), it can be seen that all species exhibit similar reductions in 5-HT at comparable combined brain levels, even though the doses administered may be very different. Thus, there is a reduction of approximately 90% in the mouse and cynomolgus monkey at approximately the same brain drug concentration (50 μM) despite a 4 times higher dose (40 mg kg^{-1}) in the mouse. Therefore, the differences in the apparent response of the species, as reported by several authors for a number of substituted phenylethylamines, is most probably due to differences in kinetics and not necessarily due to differences in sensitivity. Mennini (pers. comm.) has shown in isolated synaptosomes that for dexfenfluramine there are few species differences in effect on 5-HT uptake and release, and preliminary studies in humans have shown that the same is true. Any differences which do occur are most likely because of differences in the rate of formation of the more active metabolite, dexnorfenfluramine. Indeed, at lower levels, this becomes more important, but for simplicity it is not discussed here.

KINETIC–DYNAMIC MODELLING

Since there is little apparent animal species differences in response, it can be assumed that a comparable effect would occur at a given brain level in humans. It should therefore be possible to predict what changes in 5-HT levels could be

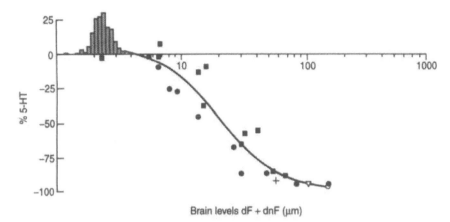

Fig. 5. Comparison of brain levels of serotonin (5-HT) and combined levels of dexfenfluramine (df) and dexnorfenfluramine (dnf) in various species and the frequency distribution of drug levels calculated from human clinical studies. Non-linear curve-fitted parameters obtained from sigmoidal E_{max} model (Campbell, 1990), where C is brain concentration.

$$\%5\text{-HT} = \frac{107 \times C^{118}}{20^{118} + C^{118}} + 6.4$$

Key: ■, mouse; ●, rat; ▽, rhesus monkey; +, cynomolgus monkey; ○, squirrel monkey.

expected during therapy. The data shown in Fig. 5 were analysed using a non-linear Michaelis–Menten receptor-based interaction model to relate brain levels of combined drug and metabolite, assuming comparable activity and changes in 5-HT. Although data shown here only relate to 5-HT, similar results are found for the metabolite 5-HIAA. A sigmoidal E_{max} model (Campbell, 1990) adequately fitted the data from all the animal species ($R^2 =$ 0.92) and the computed coefficients of this model are shown. The range and frequency distribution of human brain levels calculated from the Index study (assuming a brain-to-plasma ratio of 8) are also indicated and it can be seen visually that these concentrations are lower than those producing marked reductions in 5-HT. More precision can be obtained by substituting the mean (1.2 μM) and maximum compared brain levels attained (4.8 μM) into the equation and calculating the change in 5-HT. Thus, on average, the likely brain level of 5-HT in humans marginally increases by 5.8% at therapeutic doses, whilst at the highest measured concentration in one subject, it could be expected to be reduced fractionally by -0.9%. It could be argued that we have used the monkey-corrected value to calculate the human brain levels, and if this assumption is invalid, then we are underestimating the potential risk. If we now calculate the worst case scenario and use the uncorrected values, the mean levels still produce an increase in 5-HT, but somewhat smaller, 4.2%, whilst at the highest level, there is a small reduction, 15%, a value which in other animals is known to return to baseline in a few days. Thus, there appears to be little chance that dexfenfluramine could produce the degree of 5-HT reduction in humans observed when the animals are overdosed. This also confirms the findings in animals that reductions in 5-HT are not necessary to produce an activity, and the high doses that have been used in the past to obtain ED_{50} or more, have little justification in the therapeutic use of the drug. In humans, a daily reduction of more than 50% of food intake is unsustainable without clinical problems.

SAFETY MARGINS

To be able to assess the full safety of a compound, it is necessary to compare the dose or level of the drug which is used therapeutically in humans with that which produces an undesirable effect in animals. For many compounds, the level at the active site is not known and many uncertainty factors are included in this calculation. For dexfenfluramine, there is now the opportunity, perhaps for the first time for any drug acting on the CNS, to calculate discrete exposure safety margins. Depletion of 5-HT in itself cannot be considered as being a manifestation of toxicity, but long term depletion for several months cannot be explained, and although there are no functional correlates, this can be taken as an unwanted effect. In the long-term rat study published in this volume (see Moore, this volume), it has been shown that at a dosage of 8 mg kg day^{-1} the brain levels of 5-HT return to baseline, this can be considered as a no effect level (NOEL). At the highest dose employed, although there was a gradual increase in the depressed 5-HT levels, they had not returned to baseline after 1 year, and this can be considered as the lowest effective level (LOEL). A comparison of the mean human therapeutic and rat brain levels at the NOEL show a difference of 25-fold, whilst at the LOEL, there is an exposure margin of 68. Again, the worst case scenario must be examined and, for the one individual who may have had extreme levels, the difference becomes 6 at the NOEL and 17 at the LOEL.

But how does this compare with other drugs and what is the normal acceptable margin of safety? Of course, these considerations will depend on the type of toxicity and the importance of the disease. Thus, low margins of safety for anti-cancer or AIDS agents are more acceptable than those obtained for drugs which are used, for example, for the treatment of headaches. Recently, Contrera *et al.* (1995) published a list of exposure margins for drugs in development and which had been examined by the US Food and Drug

Administration (FDA). The safety margins based on plasma drug levels in these 35 compounds ranged from 0.11 for a non-steroidal anti-inflammatory drug (NSAID) to greater than 1000 for an antiviral with a median of 4.3. Although there are no hard and fast rules, generally margins above 5 are acceptable, and above 10 there is little concern. Thus, for dexfenfluramine, which produces a neurochemical change with no functional correlate and no human behavioural changes, is indicated as the only long-term treatment of obesity, a life-threatening disease, and which has a safety margin in excess of 10, it must be concluded that this drug is safe to be used in humans.

SUMMARY

Despite the fact that for more than 30 years fenfluramine and its isomer, dexfenfluramine, have been used throughout the world and there have been no consistently reported CNS adverse effects indicative of neurotoxicity, the results from the high-dose studies undertaken in animals have been of legitimate concern. The work briefly reviewed here exemplifies how a logical approach can resolve such a problem. The reductions in 5-HT can occur in all species if given high enough doses, but in themsleves are not indicative of neurodegeneration and functional changes. Indole levels do return to baseline, but the rate of return is proportional to the initial reduction. Doses cannot be used as a species comparator because of differences in kinetics and metabolism and brain levels across the species must be compared with the neurochemical changes. From MRS and long-term clinical studies in patients, it has been possible to compare mean and maximum drug levels in human brains and, perhaps for the first time, use mathematical models to calculate the likely changes in indoles at therapeutic doses. These clearly indicate that the majority of patients will have little change in 5-HT brain levels and only at the extremes is there a small reduction which, from animal studies, would return to baseline within a few days. Similarly, these calculations have shown a good safety margin which is higher than many other drugs where no long-term human safety data are available. In conclusion, this work has brought together a variety of scientific disciplines to confirm the safety of dexfenfluramine in humans.

Acknowledgements

We would like to thank the many scientists who, over the years, have contributed to the results presented here, including B. Guy-Grand, S. Garattini, B. Moore, N. Laudignon, C. Nathan, J. Duhault, Y. Rolland, N. Marchant, B. Gordon, B. Guardiola, M. Rebuffé-Scrive, B. Sandage and D. Gammans.

REFERENCES

Baumgarten G, Garattini S, Lorens S, Wurtman R (1992) Dexfenfluramine and neurotoxicity (Letters). *Lancet* **339**: 359.

Bendotti C, Baldessari S, Ehret M, Tarizzo G, Samanin R (1993) Effect of d-fenfluramine and 5,7-dihydroxytryptamine on the levels of tryptophan hydroxylase and its mRNA in rat brain. *Mol Brain Res* **19**: 257–261.

Boxembaum H (1982) Interspecies scaling, allometry, physiological time and the ground plan of pharmacokinetics. *J Pharmacokin Biopharmacol* **10**: 201–227.

Caccia S, Ballabio M, Guiso G, Rocchetti M (1982) Species differences in the kinetics and metabolism of fenfluramine isomers. *Arch Int Pharmacodyn* **258**: 15–28.

Caccia S, Anelli M, Ferrarese A, Fracasso C, Garattini S (1993) The role of d-norfenfluramine in the indole-depleting effect of d-fenfluramine in the rat. *Eur J Pharmacol* **233**: 71–77.

Campbell DB (1990) The use of kinetic–dynamic interactions in the evaluation of drugs. *Psychopharmacology* **100**: 433–450.

Campbell DB (1991) Dexfenfluramine: An overview of its mechanism of action. *Rev Contemp Pharmacother* **2**: 93–113.

Campbell DB (1995) Sizing up the problem of exposure extrapolation: New directions in allometric scaling. In: Thomas H, Hess R and Waechter F (eds) *Toxicology of Compounds*, Taylor & Francis, London: 45–58.

Carlton J, Rowland NE (1989) Long term actions of d-fenfluramine in two rat models of obesity. I. Sustained reductions in body weight and adiposity without depletion of brain serotonin. *Int J Obesity* **13**: 825–847.

Christensen JD, Yurgelun-Todd DA, English CD, Gruber S, Cohen BM, Renshaw F (1995) Measurement of human brain dexfenfluramine concentration by ^{19}F MR spectroscopy. *International Society of Magnetic Resonance, 3rd Scientific Meeting & Exhibition*, Nice, France, 19–25 August, Abstract No. 1852.

Clineschmidt B V, Zacchei A G, Totaro J A, Pfleuger A B, McGuffin J C, Wishousky TI (1978) Fenfluramine and Brain Serotonin. *Ann N Y Acad Sci* **305**: 221–241.

Contrera JF, Jacobs AC, Prasanna HR, Mehta M, Schmidt WJ, De George JA (1995) Systemic exposure-based alternative to the maximum tolerated dose for carcinogenicity studies of human therapeutics. *J Am Coll Toxic* **14**(1): 1–10.

Fleisher MR, Campbell DB (1969) Fenfluramine overdosage. *Lancet*, 1306–1307.

Fracasso C, Guiso G, Confalonieri S, Bergami A, Garattini S, Caccia S (1995) . Depletion and time course of recovery of brain serotonin after repeated subcutaneous dexfenfluramine in the mouse: A comparison with the rat. *Neuropharmacology* **34**(12): 1653–1659.

Fuller RW, Snoddy HD, Robertson DW (1988) Mechanisms of effects of d-fenfluramine on brain serotonin metabolism in rats: uptake inhibition versus release. Pharmacol. Biochem. & Behav **30**: 715–721.

Guy-Grand B, Crepaldi G, Lefebvre P, Appelbaum M, Gries A, Turner P (1989) International trial of long-term dexfenfluramine in obesity. *The Lancet*, 1142–1145.

Hoebel B, Schwartz D, West HL, Mark GP, Hernandez, L (1991) Serotonin micro dialysis in the hypothalamus during feeding, learned taste aversion, fluoxetine, fenfluramine and tryptophan. *Monit Mol Neurosci Proc Int Conf. In vivo methods* **5th**: 212–215.

Holmes T, Gordon B (1989) Analysis of overdosage post mortem samples for dl-fenfluramine and norfenfluramine. *Internal Servier Report* No. 89–768–002.

Invernizzi R, Berettera C, Garattini S, Samanin R (1986) D- and l-isomers of fenfluramine differ markedly in their interaction with brain serotonin and catecholamines in the rat. *Eur J Pharmacol* **120**: 9–15.

Johnson MP, Nichols DE (1990) Comparative Serotonin Neurotoxicity of the Stereo-isomers of Fenfluramine and Norfenfluramine. *Pharmacol Biochem Behav* **36**: 105–109.

Kalia M (1991) Prolonged administration of d-fenfluramine is not associated with any long lasting effect on neocortical 5-HT innervation. *21st Annual Meeting of The Society for Neuroscience Abstract Book*, p. 1439. Society for Neuroscience, Washington D.C.

Kalia M (1992) Dexfenfluramine when administered orally in doses in considerable excess of the human therapeutic dose, produces no ultrastructural or axonal transport changes in raphe serotonergic neurons of the rat. *Soc Neurosci Abstr* **18**(1): 749.

Kalia M (1996) The significance of fenfluramine/dexfenfluramine-induced neuro-chemical changes: 1976–1996. *This volume*.

Kalia M, O'Malley N (1993) Brain serotonergic system shows no changes in axonal transport or ultrastructure following short and long term treatment with dexfen-fluramine: A comparison with know serotonergic neurotoxins parachloramphet-amine and 5–7 DHT. *ISN Meeting*, Montpellier.

Karson CN, Newton JEO, Mohanakrishnan P, Sprigg J, Komoroski A (1992) Fluoxetine and trifluoperazine in human brain: A ^{19}F-nuclear magnetic resonance spectroscopy study. *Psychiat Res Neuroimaging* **45**: 95–104.

Kleven MS, Schuster CR, Seiden LS (1988) Effects of depletion of brain serotonin by repeated fenfluramine on neurochemical and anorectic effects of acute fenflur-amine. *J Pharmacol Exp Ther* **246**(3): 822–828.

Lorens S, Hata N, George M, Holne G (1993) Functional and neurochemical effects of the substituted amphetamines: Comparison with 6-hydroxydopamine (6-OHDA) and 5,7-dihydroxytryptamine (5,7-DHT). *International Society for Neuro-chemistry Meeting*, 19–20 August, Nice.

Marchant NC, Breen MA, Wallace D, Bass S, Taylor AR, Ings RMJ, Campbell DB (1992) Comparative biodisposition and metabolism in mouse, rat, dog and man. *Xenobiotica* **12**: 1251–1266.

McCann U, Hatzidimitriou G, Ridenour A, Fischer C, Yuan J, Katz J, Ricaurte G (1994) Dexfenfluramine and Serotonin Neurotoxicity: Further Preclinical Evi-dence that Clinical Caution is Indicated. *J Pharmacol Exp Ther* **269**: 792–798.

Mennini T, Bizzi A, Caccia S, Codegoni A, Fracasso C, Frittoli E, Guiso G, Padura IN, Taddei C, Uslenghi A, Garattini S (1991) Comparative studies on the anorectic activity of d-fenfluramine in mice, rats, and guinea pigs. *Naunyn-Schmiedeberg's Arch Pharmacol* **343**: 483–490.

Molliver DC, Molliver ME (1990) Anatomic evidence for a neurotoxic effect of (+/−)fenfluramine upon serotonergic projections in the rat. *Brain Res* **511, 1**: 165–168.

O'Callaghan JP (1996) Reactive gliosis as an indicator of neurotoxicity. *This volume*.

O'Callaghan JP, Miller DB (1994) Neurotoxicity profiles of substituted amphetamines in the C57/BL/6J mouse. *JPET* **270**(2): 741–751.

Oliver L, Boistesselin R, Duhault J (1978) Lack of histological neurotoxicity during fenfluramine treatment in the rat. *Pharmacology* **6**: 463.

Raleigh MJ, Brammer GL, Ritvo ER, Geller E, McGuire MT, Yuwiler A (1986) Effects of chronic fenfluramine on blood serotonin cerebrospinal fluid metabolites, and behavior in monkeys. *Psychopharmacology* **90**: 503–508.

Rattray M, Wotherspoon G, Savery D, Baldessari S, Marden C, Priestley JV, Bendotti C (1994) Chronic d-fenfluramine decreases serotonin transporter messenger RNA expression in dorsal raphe nucleus. *Eur J Pharmacol Mol Pharmacol* **268**: 439–442.

Renshaw PF, Guimaraes AR, Fava M, Rosenbaum JF, Pearlman JD, Flood JG, Puopolo PR, Clancy K, Gonzalez RG (1992) Accumulation of Fluoxetine and Norfluoxetine in Human Brain during Therapeutic Administration. Am. J. Psychiat **149**(11): 1592.

Rose S, Hunt S, Collins P, Hidmarsh JG and Jenner P (1996) Repeated administration of escalating high doses of dexfenfluramine does not produce morphological evidence for neurotoxicity in the cortex of rats. *Neurodegeneration* **5**: (in press).

Schmidt CJ (1992) L-Dopa potentiates the neurotoxicity of some amphetamine analogues. *Ann NY Acad Sci* **648**: 343–344.

Schwartz D, Hernandez L, Hoebel BG (1989) Fenfluramine administered systematically or locally increases extracellular serotonin in the lateral hypothalamus as measured by microdialysis. *Brain Res* **482**: 261–270.

Sotelo C, Zamora A (1979) Lack of Morphological Changes in the Neurons of the B-9 Group in Rats Treated with Fenfluramine. *Curr Med Res Opin* **6**(1): 55–62.

Sotelo C (1991) Immunohistochemical study of short- and long-term effects of dl-fenfluramine on the serotonergic innervation of the rat hippocampal formation. *Brain Res* **541**: 309–326.

Trouvin J-H, Gardier AM, Chanut E, Pages N, Jacquot C (1993) Time course of brain serotonin after cessation of long-term fluoxetine treatment in the rat. *Life Sci* **52**: PL187–192.

Zaczek R, Battaglia G, Culp S, Appel NM, Contrera JF, De Souza EB (1990) Effects of repeated fenfluramine administration on indices of monoamine function in rat brain: Pharmacokinetic, dose response, regional specificity and time course data. *J Pharmacol Exp Ther* **253**: 104–112.

Part III

Redux™: Therapeutic Efficacy

Overview of the Clinical Data

Bobby W. Sandage, Jr

Interneuron Pharmaceuticals, Inc., Lexington, MA 01273, USA

Obesity is a major health problem. Several recent studies have shown that even modest amounts of weight loss provide meaningful improvement in mortality and morbidity (Goldstein, 1992; Manson *et al.*, 1990). Very few treatment options are available that produce weight loss and sustained maintenance of the weight loss. Dexfenfluramine, a serotonergic agent, has the ability to produce weight loss and sustained maintenance of the weight loss with continued treatment (Finer *et al.*, 1989; Guy-Grand *et al.*, 1989; Noble, 1990).

A recent review of the efficacy and safety data for dexfenfluramine in 19 double-blind, placebo-controlled clinical trials was conducted (Sandage *et al.*, 1994). A total of 2297 patients were included in these placebo-controlled studies ($n = 1159$ dexfenfluramine-treated patients and $n = 1138$ placebo-treated patients). The mean age was 41 years and 82% were females in both treatment groups. Dexfenfluramine patients averaged 151% of their ideal body weight compared with 153% for placebo patients. Mean body mass index (BMI) was 34.2 kg m^{-2} for dexfenfluramine-treated patients compared with 34.6 kg m^{-2} for placebo-treated patients. Mean baseline weights were 93 kg for dexfenfluramine-treated patients and 94 kg for placebo-treated patients.

Studies ranged in duration from 3 months (16 studies), to 6 months (two studies: Finer *et al.*, 1989; Noble, 1990) and 12 months (one study: Guy-Grand *et al.*, 1989). Only two of these 19 studies did not include a prescribed diet; most included a 1200–1600 kcal day^{-1} diet. Average weight loss ranged from -10.2 to -2.6 kg for dexfenfluramine-treated patients and -6.6 to a gain of $+1.3$ kg for placebo (Fig. 1). Only one of the 19 trials failed to show a statistically significant difference in favour of dexfenfluramine between treatment groups. In all of the longer-term studies, a significant difference in weight loss between treatment groups was maintained for 6 and 12 months of treatment.

Obesity Management and Redux^{TM}
ISBN 0-12-518170-1

B. W. Sandage

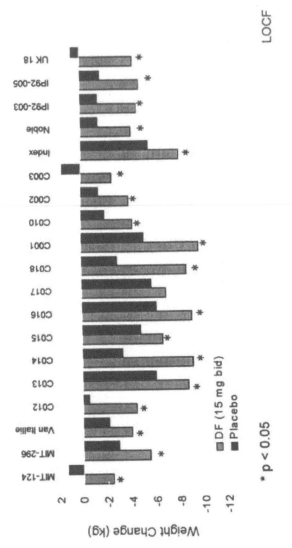

Fig. 1. Effect of dexfenfluramine in placebo-controlled weight loss trials.

In addition to the measurement of weight loss in terms of absolute weight change or per cent weight change, another way of evaluating efficacy assessed the percentage of patients attaining a specific weight loss goal or the percentage of patients that achieve weight loss in several predetermined categories (categorical analysis). In the 12-month study (Guy-Grand *et al.*, 1989), 64% of the patients treated with dexfenfluramine lost ⩾5% of their initial weight compared with only 43% of the placebo-treated patients; 40% of dexfenfluramine patients lost ⩾10% of their initial weight compared with 21% of placebo patients; 21% dexfenfluramine patients achieved ⩾15% weight loss compared with 10% placebo patients. The two 6-month studies demonstrated that 36% and 46% of the dexfenfluramine-treated patients lost ⩾5% of their initial body weight compared with 5% and 19% of the placebo-treated patients, respectively (Finer *et al.*, 1989; Noble, 1990).

For most drug therapies, markers do not exist that enable clinicians to predict *a priori* therapeutic success. By retrospectively evaluating a host of factors, a highly significant specific predictor for the therapeutic success with dexfenfluramine was identified. A patient was highly likely to lose at least 10% of their initial body weight by the end of 1 year if they lost at least 4 lb (2 kg) of body weight within the first 4 weeks of treatment. This simple therapeutic trial allows the clinician to seek alternative therapy for a patient who is not likely to respond to dexfenfluramine therapy (Sandage *et al.*, 1995).

Short-term (<4 months), placebo-controlled, double-blind studies have provided evidence that dexfenfluramine does not adversely affect glycaemia, lipid profile, or blood pressure control in obese patients. Some short-term studies have suggested that weight loss with dexfenfluramine may be associated with a reduction in hyperglycaemia in obese diabetic patients, a reduction in blood pressure in obese hypertensive patients, and improvement in the lipid profile in obese hyperlipidaemic patients (Guy-Grand *et al.*, 1989; Tauber-Lassen *et al.*, 1990; Willey *et al.*, 1992; Stewart *et al.*, 1993; Bremer *et al.*, 1994; Willey *et al.*, 1994).

The most common adverse events associated with dexfenfluramine treatment were diarrhoea, asthenia, dry mouth and somnolence. These tended to dissipate over time, with continued therapy. Adverse events leading to discontinuation occurred in 6.9% of the dexfenfluramine-treated patients and 5.2% of the placebo-treated patients (Sandage *et al.*, 1994). The most common events associated with discontinuation included asthenia, insomnia and depression.

In summary, dexfenfluramine, as an adjunct to diet, was found to produce significantly more weight loss than placebo for up to 1 year. The safety and effectiveness beyond 1 year have not been determined at this time. Finally, the common adverse events are generally mild and transient.

REFERENCES

Bremer JM, Scott RS, Lintort CJ (1994) Dexfenfluramine reduces cardiovascular risk factors. *Int J Obesity* **18**: 199–205.

Finer N, Finer S, Naoumova R (1989) Prolonged use of a very low calorie diet (Cambridge diet) in massively obese patients attending an obesity clinic: Safety, efficacy and additional benefit from dexfenfluramine. *Int J Obesity* **13**: 91–93.

Goldstein DF (1992) Beneficial health effects of modest weight loss. *Int J Obesity* **16**: 397–416

Guy-Grand B, Apfelbaum M, Crepaldi G, Gries A, Lefebvre P, Turner P (1989) International trial of long-term dexfenfluramine in obesity. *Lancet*: 1142–1145.

Kolanowski J, Younis L, Vanbutsele R, Detry J (1992) Effect of dexfenfluramine treatment on body weight, blood pressure and noradrenergic activity in obese hypertensive patients. *Eur J Clin Pharmacol* **42**: 599–606.

Lucas CP, Sandage BW (1995) Treatment of obese patients with dexfenfluramine: A multi-center, placebo-controlled study. *Am J Ther* **2**: 962–967.

Manson J, Colditz G, Stampfer M *et al*. (1990) A prospective study of obesity and risk of coronary heart disease in women. *New Engl J Med* **322**: 883–889.

McTavish D, Heel R (1992) Dexfenfluramine: A review of its pharmacological properties and therapeutic potential in obesity. *Drugs* **43**: 713–733.

Noble RE (1990) A six-month study of the effects of dexfenfluramine on partially successful dieters. *Curr Ther Res* **47**: 612–619.

Sandage BW, Loar SB, Laudignon N (1994) Review of Dexfenfluramine Efficacy and Safety. *Int J Obesity*, Vol 18, Suppl 2, p 135, August.

Sandage BW, Loar SB, Cooper GL (1995). Predictor of Therapeutic Success with Dexfenfluramine. *Obesity Res* **3**(Suppl. 3): O122.

Stewart GO, Stein GR, Davis TM, Findlater P (1993) Dexfenfluramine in Type II Diabetes: Effects on Weight and Diabetes Control. *Med J Austral*, Vol. 158, p167–168.

Tauber-Lassen E, Damsbo P, Henriksen JE, Palmvig B, Beck-Nielsen H (1990) Improvement of glycemic control and weight loss in type 2 (non-insulin-dependent) diabetics after one year of dexfenfluramine treatment. *Diabetologia* **33**: A124.

Willey KA, Molyneaux LM, Yue DK (1994) Obese Patients with Type II Diabetes Poorly Controlled by Insulin and Metformin: Effects of Adjunctive Dexfenfluramine Therapy on Glycemic Control. *Diabetic Med* 701–704.

Willey KA, Molyneaux LM, Overland JE, Yue DK (1992) The effects of Dexfenfluramine on blood glucose control in patients with type 2 diabetes. *Diabetic Med* **9**: 341–43.

INDEX Study: Weight Data and Effects on Risk Factors and Comorbidities

Bernard Guy-Grand

*Department of Medicine and Nutrition, Hôtel-Dieu Hospital, Paris,
75181 Cedex, France*

The Index (International Dexfenfluramine study) (Guy-Grand *et al.*, 1989) was the first large controlled trial of an anti-obesity drug designed on a 1-year basis to test the feasibility and clinical relevance of prolonged use of dexfenfluramine (Redux^{TM}) in the management of this harmful chronic disease, which has an increasing prevalence. This study substantiated an in-depth evolution of the concepts underlying the pharmacotherapy of obesity (Guy-Grand, 1987). The data presented 3 years later by M. Weintraub on a combination of phentermine and fenfluramine (Weintraub *et al.*, 1992) confirmed the value of this approach, which has been very recently recognized by the US Food and Drug Administration (FDA).

The Index study was a multicentre randomized placebo-controlled double-blind trial, designed on an intention-to-treat basis, which included 822 obese patients (from 120% to 306% ideal body weight) of either sex. A 15 mg dose twice daily of dexfenfluramine (dF) was prescribed for 404 of the subjects, while 418 were prescribed a placebo (P). All patients were also prescribed a diet because it was judged unethical to maintain patients under placebo alone for longer than 1 year.

BODY WEIGHT CONTROL

The main results can be summarized as follows:

(1) *Reinforcement of the adherence to long-term weight-lowering programme.* In keeping with the well-known poor compliance of obese patients to dietary restriction, helping them to cope better with dietary restriction would

appear to be important. At 12 months it appeared that significantly more patients ($p < 0.002$) had withdrawn from P than from dF, representing 45% and 37% of the cohorts, respectively. Dissatisfaction with the weight loss was the only reason more frequently reported in the P than in the dF group (84 vs 49, $p < 0.02$), accounting for almost all the excess of withdrawals in the P group.

(2) *Increase in the number of patients achieving a significant weight loss.* The intention to treat analysis which accounts for all patients who achieve a given target weight is the more clinically relevant and probably the less biased evaluation of the efficacy of any treatment. When calculated in the cohort of patients completing the study, 52% vs 30% of the patients had lost more than 10% of their starting weight and 48% vs 27% had lost more than 10 kg at 12 months in the dF and P cohorts, respectively ($p < 0.001$). When considering the patients who entered the study and regarding drop-outs as non-losers, the corresponding figures were 34.9% vs 17% and 32.4% vs 15% ($p < 0.001$). Among the predictors of such targets weight loss ≤2% at 1 month and/or ≥10% at 4 months had the best negative and positive (respectively) predictive value (Guy-Grand *et al.*, 1996). Therefore dF allowed twice as many patients to achieve a weight loss, the magnitude of which is now considered as a medically acceptable target for improving significantly health risk factors and some diseases associated with obesity.

(3) *Increase in average weight loss.* Comparison of mean weight loss in the residual cohorts has the disadvantages of mixing weight losers and non-losers and of being largely dependent on the drop-out rate; it overestimated weight loss in the P cohort, which contained an excess of withdrawn patients. Even with these drawbacks, the dF completers had lost significantly ($p < 0.001$) more weight after 12 months (9.82 ± 0.49 kg) than the P completers (7.15 ± 0.49 kg), i.e. 10.26% and 7.18% of starting weight. This difference could be estimated as a weak one but the extra weight loss of dF patients was 52% over that of P patients. The assay of plasma dF and of its active metabolite d-norfenfluramine allowed us to demonstrate a positive correlation ($r = 0.52$, $p < 0.002$) between weight loss and their combinated plasma levels (unpublished data). It is important to note that the significant weight loss achieved by the P cohort was likely to result from the combined effects of placebo, associated diet and supportive management by the investigators, and could be favourably compared with those of diet alone.

(4) *Maintenance of efficacy over 1 year.* The goal and the major challenge in the treatment of obesity is helping patients to maintain totally or partially their initial weight loss and to prevent the very high rate of relapse (Wadden *et al.*, 1989). A weight plateau was reached with dF after 6 months (an evolution

typical of that observed with all the procedures aimed at losing weight), with maintenance of the weight loss up to 12 months. Those in the placebo group regained weight significantly ($p < 0.05$). When dF was withdrawn after completion of the study, a rapid weight gain occurred within 2 months. During the 6-month plateau the action of the drug was not to promote additional weight loss but to prevent weight regain.

(5) *Tolerance and safety*. The only symptoms that were significantly more frequent in dF than in P patients were tiredness, diarrhoea, dry mouth, polyuria and drowsiness, most often recorded during the first or second month of treatment. They must be considered as the true side effects of the drug. No major hazards imputable to dF were reported in the Index study.

ACTION ON RISK FACTORS AND CO-MORBIDITIES

From a medical viewpoint, it is clear that weight loss and its maintenance cannot be considered as targets *per se*: a concomitant improvement of metabolic or haemodynamic endpoints must be documented in order to assess the benefit/risk or the benefit/costs ratios.

Glucose metabolism and non-insulin dependent diabetes (NIDDM)

Unpublished data from Index indicated that on average fasting blood glucose in mostly non-diabetic patients significantly decreased both in P and dF cohorts (from 5.5 to 5.3 mmol l^{-1}, $p = 0.002$ and from 5.7 to 5.3 mmol l^{-1}, $p < 0.001$ respectively), with no significant treatment $\times$ time interaction. This decrease was obtained by the sixth month and maintained up to the twelfth.

Plasma lipids

Unpublished data from Index indicated a significant and sustained decrease in total plasma cholesterol and triglycerides both in dF and P group with no treatment $\times$ time interaction. In the subgroup of hypercholesterolaemic patients (total cholesterol > 6.5 mmol l^{-1}), large decrease in total cholesterol was observed at the end of the study: 7.3 to 6.5 mmol l^{-1} in the dF group ($p < 0.001$) and 7.4 to 7 mmol l^{-1} ($p = 0.002$) in the P group. Again there was no significant treatment $\times$ time interaction but a significant ($p < 0.002$) drug effect was obtained with average total cholesterol reverted to normal in the dF group. This differential effect was likely to be due to the fact that dF patients have lost more weight (9.9 kg vs 6.36 kg).

Blood pressure

From the Index study, we recently reported (Guy-Grand *et al.*, 1994) the time course of blood pressure in the 214 and 230 (P and dF groups, respectively) obese subjects whose blood pressure measurements were available from baseline up to 12 months. Significant decreases were observed: 7.42 ± 0.6 and 8.75 ± 0.9 mmHg for systolic blood pressure (SBP) and 4.12 ± 0.6 and 5.51 ± 0.6 mmHg for diastolic blood pressure (DBP) in P and dF groups, respectively. Although no significant treatment $\times$ time interaction was observed, it was apparent that both SBP and DBP were longer in the dF group at each time point (except baseline) and also that the major part of this decrease was achieved by the second month. In the subset of hypertensive patients (DBP > 95 mmHg at the start), mean DBP decreased more rapidly in the dF group (treatment $\times$ time interaction $p < 0.05$) so that significantly more patients did not remain hypertensive by the second month of treatment (30.8% vs 50%, P vs dF). Also DBP was stabilized from the second to the twelfth month with dF and tended to increase with P after the sixth month. When adjusting on weight loss (linear covariance analysis) the fall in DBP was larger in the dF group at the second month of treatment by 5.2 mmHg ($p < 0.002$), thus suggesting a weight independent effect of dF on blood pressure.

Taken together all these data indicate that not only during the weight lowering period but more importantly in the long-term, sustained weight loss of moderate importance is able to induce stable improvements in metabolic and haemodynamic risk factors and diseases associated with obesity. Dexfenfluramine, which clearly increased the number of patients responding to weight lowering programmes would appear to be well suited in hypertensive, hyperlipidaemic or diabetic obese patients, particularly when classical treatments of these diseases do not allow them to be controlled.

HOW TO USE DEXFENFLURAMINE

Since obesity is a chronic disease and current treatments mostly palliative, only able to alleviate the symptom but not to cure it, the question of long-term (eventually lifelong) pharmacotherapy is obviously raised. To engage a patient in any lifelong treatment, however, requires serious consideration. The use of drugs should be restricted to those who are at risk as a result of their obesity, or to those with medical conditions that will be ameliorated by sustained weight loss (e.g. diabetes, hypertension, rheumatology and respiratory disorders).

The clinical data obtained in Index (and other trials) clearly indicated that this drug should be seriously considered in the therapeutic strategies to be developed for the management of many obese patients, in addition to diet that is to be tried first. Indications for dF could be the following:

(1) failure to adhere to a reasonable diet;
(2) stress induced snacking;
(3) high blood pressure, NIDDM, hyperlipidaemia, excess abdominal body fat often associated in the so-called Syndrome X, and/or a familial history of these diseases;
(4) maintenance of body weight stability in rapidly gaining patients and/or prevention of relapse following weight loss obtained by other non-invasive procedures.

Since early failure seems to predict longer-term outcome, patients might be started on dF. If efficient, the prescription should be maintained. Its duration might be adapted to the specific outcome of each patient.

It must be emphasized, however, that the prescription of drugs must not dodge a thorough evaluation of the underlying problems nor prevent other types of useful interventions. Also their long-term use must be restricted to those patients at risk and not used for cosmetic purposes. Dexfenfluramine must be included in multifaceted long-term management programmes and strategies, individually tailored and including simultaneously or sequentially diets, behaviour modifications and physical exercise.

REFERENCES

Guy-Grand B (1987) A new approach to the treatment of obesity: a discussion. In: Wurtman RJ and Wurtman JJ (eds) *Human Obesity. Ann NY Acad Sci* **499**: 313–317.

Guy-Grand B, Apfelbaum M, Crepaldi G, Gries A, Lefebvre P, Turner P (1989) International trial of long-term Dexfenfluramine in obesity. *Lancet* **ii**: 1142–1144.

Guy-Grand B, Apfelbaum M, Crepaldi G, Gries A, Lefebvre P, Turner P (1994) Dexfenfluramine lowers blood pressure independently of weight loss: Data from Index study. *Int J Obesity* **18** (suppl. 2): 48.

Guy-Grand B, Apfelbaum M, Crepaldi G, Gries A, Lefebvre P, Turner P (1996) Short-term predictors of successful weight loss with Dexfenfluramine (dF). *Int J Obesity* **20**(suppl. 4): 70.

Wadden TA, Sternberg JA, Letizia KA, Stunkard AJ, Foster GD (1989) Treatment of obesity by very low calorie diet, behavior therapy, and their combination: A five year perspective. *Int J Obesity* **13**(suppl. 2): 39–46.

Weintraub M, Sundaresan PR, Cox C (1992) Long-term weight control study. VI: Individual participant response pattern. *Clin Pharmacol Ther* **51**: 619–633.

An 18-month Study of the Effects of Dexfenfluramine on Cognitive Function in Obese American Patients

Rudolf E. Noble

Director, Cathedral Hill Obesity Clinic, San Francisco, CA 94103, USA

Dexfenfluramine has now been used extensively as an anorectic agent in an estimated 10 million people in 65 countries worldwide. This anorexiant seems to be an effective and safe medication as verified by this vast marketing population, as well as by controlled clinical trials in over 4000 patients. Nevertheless, some reports have cropped up in the literature that in some experimental animals cytological neuronal changes have been induced when the drug is administered in doses exceeding the maximum human dose. The clinical relevance of these changes is questionable and no behavioural or functional adverse effects have been observed in animals.

The purpose of this study was to determine, via a comprehensive battery of psychiatric tests, if dexfenfluramine has any subtle effects on the CNS in *humans*. The following four psychiatric check-list tests were conducted before, during and at the end of 6 months of continuous dexfenfluramine administration and three times in the 1 year follow-up placebo period thereafter.

(1) The Profile of Mood Scale (POMS) to determine any changes in mood.
(2) The Mini Mental State (MMS) Examination to detect changes in cognition.
(3) The Center for Epidemiological Studies Depression (CES-D) test for changes in depression.
(4) The Stanford Sleepiness Scale (SSS) to detect changes in daytime sleepiness patterns

Obesity Management and Redux^{TM}
ISBN 0-12-518170-1

Figure 1 shows the design of the study. This was a randomized, double-blind, parallel, placebo-controlled study spanning 18 months. Following a 1-week selection period, the study proceeded in two phases.

The first phase was a double-blind, randomized phase for the first 6 months during which patients received either dexfenfluramine 15 mg b.i.d. or matching placebo b.i.d. p.o.

The second phase was a single-blind placebo 'withdrawal' phase with discontinuation of dexfenfluramine and substitution of placebo for 12 months for both treatment groups. Seventy-one adult, male and female, out-patients aged between 18 and 65 years inclusive were entered into the study. These were obese patients who were chosen at the Cathedral Hill Obesity Clinic and who were between 20% and 75% above ideal body weight according to the Metropolitan Life Insurance Company Actuarial Tables, i.e. body mass index (BMI) more than 28. They had to be in excellent general physical and mental health and were not to take any medication that could affect the study. No pregnant or lactating females were allowed into the study and menstruating patients were seen, in general, on all visits during the follicular phase to avoid seeing any premenstrual mood changes.

Patients were all placed on standard calorie-restricted diets during the trial. Patients were well matched in both groups, being mostly females (about 75%) and 50%–50% black–white. About one-half of the patients completed all 18 months: 18 dexfenfluramine and 12 placebo. Weight, blood pressure, pulse, side effects and global appetite evaluation were also recorded, as shown in Fig. 1. Drug compliance was excellent, being in excess of 90%. Patients were, in addition, queried at all visits as follows:

'Since your last visit, have you felt or noticed any changes in terms of . . .?': headaches, tiredness, sleep, dreams, personal problems, sexual activities, digestion, mood, energy or impulse control.

Figure 2 shows the results at the end of the study of the POMS test, i.e. mood ratings further broken down and graded into six categories: anxiety, depression, anger, vigour, fatigue and confusion. As can be seen from this figure, there are no significant differences at the end of the 18 months, nor were there at any time during the course of this study for any of the six parameters.

Figure 3 shows the results of the effects of dexfenfluramine on cognition as detected by the MMS Exam scores. Shown here are the scores on the completers at each visit. Scores for all patients stayed above 25, well within the normal range, and did not differ between placebo and dexfenfluramine-treated patients during treatment or in the 12 months of placebo substitution using either the observed cases or completer data.

Figure 4 shows the results of the Center of Epidemiological Studies Depression (CES-D) scores. Data for the completers at each time point are shown in this diagram. There are no dexfenfluramine or placebo differences in the CES-D scores either during treatment or in the 12 month placebo

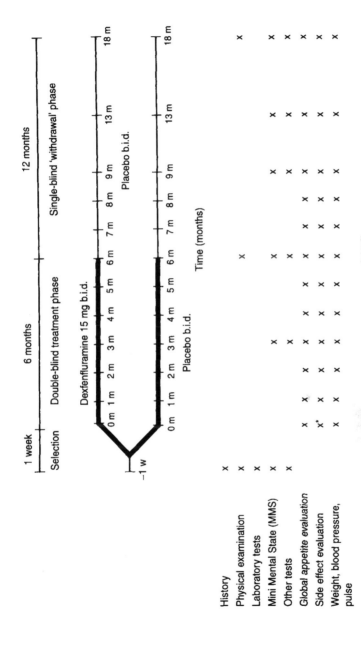

Fig. 1. Study design. The asterisk indicates that an enquiry of complaints of any symptoms was made before the start of the study.

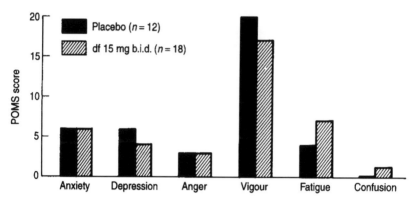

Fig. 2.   Effect of dexfenfluramine (dF) on mood 12 months after the double-blind phase.

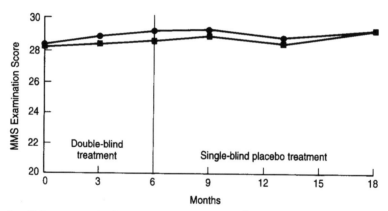

Fig. 3.   Effects of dexfenfluramine on cognition. ——●——, placebo ($n = 12$); ——■——, dexfenfluramine 15 mg b.i.d. ($n = 18$).

substitution phase using the observed cases or completer data. For reference, CES-D scores on the 21-item version would average about 35 in patients with Major Depression as diagnosed by clinical interview.

Figure 5 shows the scores for the SSS rating. Again there are no differences between treatment groups at the end of the treatment or in the placebo follow-up phase.

Also from our personal enquiries regarding any possible neuropsychiatric changes, for example sexual activities, impulse control, mood changes, etc. we found no significant differences between the two groups. Weight loss changes and side effects were similar to those reported in previous studies.

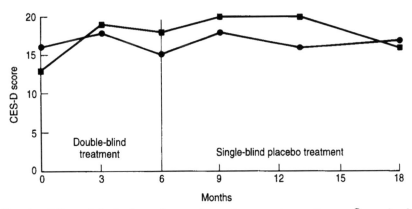

Fig. 4.   Effect of dexfenfluramine on depression symptom rating. —●—, placebo
(n = 12); —■—, dexfenfluramine 15 mg b.i.d. (n = 18).

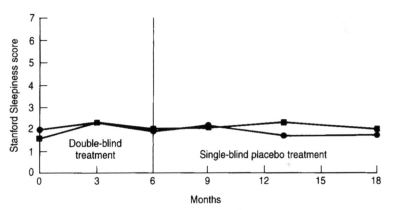

Fig. 5.   Effects of dexfenfluramine on sleep. —●—, placebo (n = 12); —■—,
dexfenfluramine 15 mg b.i.d. (n = 18).

In summary, then, we can conclude from this long-term safety study that:

dexfenfluramine, at 15 mg b.i.d., did not produce any clinically detect-
able CNS changes in mood, cognition, depression symptomatology, etc.
during 6 months of continuous treatment or during a 1-year follow-up,
i.e. a total of 18 months.

Based on these findings which comprised the results of almost 1000 CNS
queries per patient, we feel that dexfenfluramine is indeed a safe medication.

Fenfluramines, Obesity and Primary Pulmonary Hypertension: Risks and Benefits

Gerald A. Faich

President, Outcomes Research Corporation, Bala Cynwyd, PA 19004, USA
(The author has served as a consultant to Servier and Wyeth)

Introduction

Concern about a relationship between fenfluramines used for weight loss and primary pulmonary hypertension (PPH) first arose in the early part of this decade. Since then several publications, a large international case control study and regulatory hearings have addressed this concern. The present brief summary of this issue is done from a benefit/risk viewpoint.

Between 1988 and 1992, a cluster of 15 PPH cases possibly associated with fenfluramines were seen at the Hospital Antoine Beclere in Paris (Brenot *et al.*, 1993). As a result of this, Brenot and his colleagues sought regulatory action to restrict the use of fenfluramines. In part, this concern was based on the experience with aminorex, an anorectic drug which caused a distinct drug-induced epidemic of some 400 cases of PPH centred in Switzerland, Austria and Germany in 1967 and 1968 (Guntner, 1985). The aminorex epidemic came 12–18 months after the initial marketing of the drug and after approximately 500 000 individuals were exposed.

On examination of the Hospital Beclere case series, it was recognized that it would be impossible, based on such a small number of cases, to know whether these were coincidental or whether they were due to anorectic drug exposure (Abenheim *et al.*, 1994). For this reason, the International Primary Pulmonary Hypertension Study (IPPHS) was planned (Abenhaim, 1994) and conducted from 1993 to 1994. In April 1995, preliminary analyses (Abenhaim, 1995) from this case control study were provided to regulators and these

Obesity Management and Redux[TM]
ISBN 0-12-518170-1

analyses were extensively discussed by regulatory authorities in France, the USA (FDA Advisory Committees in September and November 1995) and Europe (EMEA, October 1995). The publication of some of the IPPHS results is pending at the moment (Abenhaim et al., 1996) (See Addendum on p. 104).

IPPHS

The IPPHS sought to identify all possible PPH cases seen at 220 participating cardiopulmonary referral centres located in Belgium, France, the Netherlands and the UK. When a case was preliminarily identified, study personnel were contacted and appropriate diagnostic testing was urged. All eligible cases required cardiac catheterization for measurement of pulmonary artery pressures. Data were reviewed by experts to assure that each case was truly PPH. In this way, 95 confirmed and eligible cases were identified.

As each case was identified, several controls of the same age, gender and care utilization level were sought from the same primary care physician who had cared for the case. This was done to control differential use of medication by differing physicians. When a given practitioner did not cooperate, then a physician from the same or adjacent community was sought. Both case and controls were interviewed for a variety of risk factors and exposures including use of pharmaceutical products. Afterwards, rates of exposures were determined and analysed for both cases and controls.

Initially, leaving aside seven cases exposed to extemporaneously compounded anorectic preparations and three cases of indeterminate anorectic exposure, the following results were reported from the IPPHS (Abenhaim, 1995). For the 95 cases and 355 controls, it was found that 21% of cases (20 persons) were exposed to anorectics (mainly dexfenfluramine) and only 6.5% of controls had anorectic drug exposures. The following were more likely in cases than controls (odds ratios): systemic hypertension (2.5 times), obesity (2.4 times), fenfluramines (3.8 times) and all appetite-suppressant exposure for more than 3 months (10.6 times).

Other conclusions were that:

(1) risk was not increased for anorectic drug exposure of less than 3 months;
(2) compounded anorectic preparations had a higher risk; and
(3) PPH is very rare (1.7 cases per million population per year including those with anorectic drug exposures).

Subsequent analyses (Abenhaim et al., 1996) including seven cases with compounded exposures, described 30 cases exposed to appetite suppressants. With these included, the odds risk for exposures of more than 3 months in obese individuals was calculated to be 23.

IPPHS LIMITATIONS AND INTERPRETATIONS

All observational studies, particularly those involving pharmaceuticals (Feinstein, 1985; Collet *et al.*, 1994), are subject to confounding and bias. In France and Belgium, where 81% of the PPH cases were found, there was considerable publicity (Atanassof *et al.*, 1992; Roche *et al.*, 1992; Brenot *et al.*, 1993) about a possible association between anorectics and PPH, and this must have led to heightened suspicion and referral of anorectic-exposed cases to the study hospitals. The IPPHS found that exposed cases were not less ill than non-exposed cases, but this does not fully alleviate concern about detection bias. A substantial number of PPH cases, particularly those without anorectic exposures, may never be referred or diagnosed correctly. Under-reporting of exposure to anorectic agents by controls – recall bias (Collet *et al.*, 1994) – also may have contributed to the association with anorectic agents. Even a small increase in the proportion of cases exposed and a small decrease in the controls reportedly exposed as a result of these biases could have had a substantial effect on the calculated odds ratios. A third concern is the relationship of obesity to PPH; this was not entirely resolved by the stratified and other statistical analyses done. Obesity status of case and controls was based on the maximum lifetime weight reported by cases and controls; using this, the IPPHS found an odds ratio of 1.9 for obesity. No information was collected on weight fluctuation or weight at time of anorectic drug exposure and it is plausible that the observed association with anorectics may be due, at least in part, to weight fluctuation or to weight loss itself.

It is also important to examine whether an association with PPH is particular to the fenfluramines or whether it is found with all anorectics. Of the 30 exposed cases in the IPPHS, 16 had only fenfluramine exposures, eight had no known fenfluramine exposure (mainly exposures to amphetamine-like drugs) and six had mixed exposures. With millions of exposures, the fenfluramines are, by far, the most widely used of the appetite-suppressant drugs in the study countries. This probably accounts for the preponderance of fenfluramine exposures in the study. Importantly, seven of the 18 cases with exposures of more than 3 months had used a variety of compounded preparations. These cases have a major impact on the odds ratios. Earlier analyses of the IPPHS presented to the FDA without these cases, and unadjusted for obesity, had odds ratios of only 10.6. The large effect of including compounded preparations might be due to the content of these concoctions, the characteristics of exposed patients or the study methods.

While the IPPHS does not provide conclusive evidence of a causal relationship between anorectics and PPH, nonetheless it is important to consider the absolute magnitude of the possible risk described. Due to the biases identified, using the IPPHS results provides a 'worst case' scenario. Multiplying the odds ratio times an unexposed background risk gives an absolute risk. IPPHS estimated the background rate of PPH in Belgium to be 1.7 cases per million including the exposed cases. Since 30% of cases were exposed, the unexposed background rate is about 1.2 per million. Thus, the absolute risk can be calculated to be, at most, about 28 per million person-years of exposure to anorectics (23 times 1.2). This is of the order of the death risk found for penicillin-induced anaphylaxis (Gilman *et al.*, 1985) or oral contraceptive-associated venous thromboemboli (Spitzer *et al.*, 1996) and myocardial infarction.

BENEFITS OF WEIGHT LOSS

There can be no doubt that obesity is a serious clinical and public health issue. The obesity epidemic in the US affects 30% of the population and is increasing (Kuczmarski *et al.*, 1994). Obesity is a complex, chronic disease that is resistant to treatment. Diet and exercise programmes have largely failed over the long haul. For these reasons, the adjunctive use of pharmacological agents has received renewed attention.

Obesity is now increasingly recognized as a major preventable cause of excess death. In the US it has been estimated that it contributes to 300 000 excess deaths per year, making the disease the second leading preventable cause of death after smoking (McGinnis and Foege, 1993). This is evident in examining data from the Nurses Health Study (NHS) which details mortality trends for over 115 000 nurses followed for over 16 years (Manson *et al.*, 1995). For non-smoking women, as body mass index (BMI) goes from 26 to 30.5 (a gain of about 13 kg), the NHS found all-cause mortality increases by 60–70%. This translates into an excess of about 840 lives per million per year. Most of this excess mortality is due to cardiovascular causes.

The value of using fenfluramines for treating obesity is shown by clinical trial data for dexfenfluramine. Dexfenfluramine was largely approved in the US on the basis of the Index trial which involved over 800 patients placed on diet and randomized to drug or placebo (Redux^{TM} Label; Guy-Grand *et al.*, 1989). Results showed that 74% of those taking the drug lost over 5% of their body weight and maintained this over a 12 month period of time. Importantly, there was a doubling of the proportion of the dexfenfluramine population losing 15% or more of their body weight compared with those on placebo. For patients with an initial average BMI of 32, over 60% lost 10% or more of their body weight and thus they achieved and maintained an average BMI of 29. Combining these results with NHS data on BMI-specific mortality suggests that 280 lives and 440 non-fatal myocardial infarctions and strokes could be prevented per million persons treated per year. It is against this background that the International Primary Pulmonary Hypertension Study (IPPHS) must be interpreted. It is clear that the benefits of dexfenfluramine use far exceed the theoretical risk of PPH.

SUMMARY AND DISCUSSION

There is no absolutely definitive evidence that fenfluramines cause PPH. While the international case control study (IPPHS) found a strong association between more than 3 months of exposure to dexfenfluramine and PPH based on a small number of cases, this may have been affected by differential referral and diagnosis of cases. The international study also showed an association with obesity and it is entirely possible that weight change, independent of drug exposure, may contribute to the PPH risk.

It must be emphasized that the risk of possible PPH associated with fenfluramines is rare. Indeed, the paucity of cases found by the IPPHS in Europe, despite the exposure of millions of persons to the fenfluramines, is in sharp contrast to the aminorex epidemic and provides further assurance that risk from fenfluramines must be very small. In contrast, the medical consequences of obesity, particularly cardiovascular death and disability, are very common. It can be calculated that the benefits of dexfenfluramine-induced weight loss far outweigh the possible risk of PPH.

Exposing patients to even theoretical risks can only be justified when benefits outweigh risks. Mortality improvement and other health benefits due to weight loss are likely only if weight loss is sustained. The target population most likely to benefit from weight loss agents are patients with BMIs over 30 who have failed non-pharmacological interventions. Drugs must be seen as adjunctives to diet and exercise programmes and reserved for patients who fail these measures alone. Since obesity is a chronic disease, it will be important to study further benefits and risks of weight loss agents over multiple years of drug therapy. Additionally, population-based studies to assess mortality effects must be done even though such studies will be expensive and arduous.

REFERENCES

Abenhaim L (The International Primary Pulmonary Hypertension Study Group) (1994) The International Primary Pulmonary Hypertension Study (IPPHS). *Chest* **105**(suppl): 31S–41S.

Abenhaim L (The International Primary Pulmonary Hypertension Study Group) (1995) The International Primary Pulmonary Hypertension Study (IPPHS). *Summary Report* No. 1, 7 March 1995.

Abenhaim L, Higenbottam T, Rich S (1994) International Primary Pulmonary Hypertension Study. Letter. *Br Heart J* **71**: 303–304.

Abenhaim L, Moride Y, Brenot F, *et al.* (1996) Anorexic drugs and other risk factors for primary pulmonary hypertension. Abstract, Montreal Meeting on Pulmonary Hypertension, 17 May 1996.

Atanassoff PG, Weiss BM, Schmid ER, Tornie M (1992) Pulmonary hypertension and dexfenfluramine. *Lancet* **339**: 436.

Brenot F, Herve P, Petitpretz P, Parent F *et al.* (1993) Primary pulmonary hypertension and fenfluramine use. *Br Heart J* **70**: 537–541.

Collet JP, Boisin JF, Spitzer WO (1994) Bias and confounding in pharmacoepidemiology. In: Strom BL (ed.) *Pharmacoepidemiology*. John Wiley & Sons, Chichester and New York.

Feinstein AR (1985) *Clinical Epidemiology: The Architecture of Clinical Research*. WB Saunders, Philadelphia.

Gilman AG, Goodman LS, Rall TN, Murod F (eds) (1985) *Goodman and Gilman's The Pharmacological Basis of Therapeutics*, 7th edn. MacMillan, New York.

Guntner HP (1985) Aminorex and pulmonary hypertension. *Cor Vasa* **27**: 160–171.

Guy-Grand B, Crepaldi G, Lefebvre P *et al.* (1989) International trial of long term dexfenfluramine in obesity. *Lancet* 1142–1145.

Kuczmarski RJ, Flegal KM, Campbell SM *et al.* (1994) Increasing prevalence of overweight among US adults: The National Health and Nutrition Examination Surveys, 1960 to 1991. *J Am Med Assoc* **272**: 205–211.

Manson JE, Willett WC, Stampfer MJ *et al.* (1995) Body weight and mortality among women. *New Engl J Med* **333**: 677–685.

McGinnis JM, Foege WH (1993) Actual causes of death in the United States. *J Am Med Assoc* **270**: 2207–2212.

Redux[TM] label. Wyeth Ayerst, Radnor Pa and Intercursor Pharmaceuticals Inc. Lexington Pa.

Roche N, Labrune S, Braun JM, Huchor G (1992) Pulmonary hypertension and dexfenfluramine. *Lancet* **339**: 436–7.

Spitzer WO, Lewis MA, Heinemann LA, Thorogood M *et al.* (1996) Third generation oral contraceptives and risk of venous thromboembolic disorders: An international case-control study. *Brit Med J* **312**: 83–88.

ADDENDUM

This article was prepared and submitted prior to the final publication of the IPPHS on Aug. 29, 1996 (Abenhaim L, Morida Y, Brenot F *et al.* (1996) Appetite-suppressant drugs and the risk of primary pulmonary hypertension. *New Eng. J. Med.* **335**: 609–16).

Overview of the Safety Data

N. Laudignon and M. Rebuffé-Scrive*

Institut de Recherches Internationales Servier, 6 place des Pleiades, 92415 Courbevoie, France
Servier Amérique, 22 rue Garnier 92201 Neuilly-sur-Seine, France

CLINICAL DATA BASE

General Adverse Events

These safety data have been obtained from more than 3000 obese patients treated with dexfenfluramine (dF) and were compared with similar information from more than 1100 placebo-treated patients. It is important to note that because the largest trials were also the longest, most of the patients were treated with dF for more than 6 months and over 35% were treated for 1 year.

The most commonly observed treatment-emergent adverse events occurring at a frequency equal or greater than 2% and, statistically significant from placebo-controls, were asthenia (15.8%), diarrhoea (17.5%), dry mouth (12.5%) and somnolence (7.1%). These adverse events were characterized by most of the patients as 'mild', they were transient and tended to disappear after a couple of weeks of therapy.

Because dF action is primarily in the brain, CNS adverse events were investigated more specifically. The CNS adverse events that occurred at a rate equal or greater than 1% and that were significantly different from placebo were dry mouth, somnolence and vertigo.

Discontinuations

The data on discontinuations for all placebo-controlled clinical trials obtained in 1159 dexfenfluramine-treated patients and in 1138 placebo-treated patients indicated that 67% of the dF patients completed the trials compared with

Obesity Management and Redux^{TM}
ISBN 0-12-518170-1

63% in the placebo group. Discontinuations due to an adverse event were 6.9% in the dF group and 5.2% in the placebo group. Ineffective medication was reported by 5.0% of dF-treated patients compared with 9.4% in the controls. No clinically significant differences from placebo were noticed in laboratory variables and no trends were observed in vital signs and electrocardiograms.

Medical and Safety Review of Clinical Behavioural and Cognitive Data

Discussions on neurochemical changes induced by high doses of dF have been essentially focused on the experimental findings in animals. Potential implications for human use (i.e. at therapeutic doses) have only been speculative. CNS adverse events, observed either in the controlled trials or in the postmarketing surveillance (see below), are uncommon, transient and non-specific.

For the dexfenfluramine New Drug Application, a comprehensive medical and safety review of neurological, psychometric and behavioural or cognitive data has been performed. This work was based on 17 controlled clinical trials and 55 reports in the published literature. The ratings were collected in therapeutic trials involving obese patients, or pilot therapeutic trials in other disorders, for the purpose of assessing the potential for adverse CNS consequences of dF treatment. These studies were substantial in terms of number of patients investigated, dF dose and duration of treatment, and outcome measures employed. The neuropsychopharmacological tests and rating instruments used are well established in clinical neuropsychopharmacology and are capable of detecting clinically meaningful changes in response to drug exposure. Many of these same tests are recommended by the World Health Organization (WHO) or the National Institute of Mental Health (NIMH) for evaluating neurotoxicological effects of human exposure to environmental or industrial chemicals. The review focused on human behaviours that serotonin is postulated to modulate (i.e. appetite, mood, suicidal behaviour, attention, concentration, memory) or on neurological signs.

Appetite is reduced by dF treatment, an effect consistent with its therapeutic action. After abrupt discontinuation of dF following 3 months of treatment, structured assessment of food preferences in two studies at 1 month (unpublished data) found no significant difference between dF-treated and placebo-treated patients, indicating that appetite returns to pretreatment levels promptly. The weight loss response to dF 15 mg b.i.d. in patients who regained weight in the 2 months after discontinuation of dF following 1 year of treatment (INDEX: Guy-Grand *et al.*, 1990) were evaluated and compared with results for a group of placebo-treated patients. Both groups had a similar response, indicating no lasting change in appetite resulting from 12 months of dF treatment.

Ten studies (Wurtman *et al.*, 1987, 1993; Finer *et al.*, 1989; O'Rourke *et al.*, 1989; Brzezinski *et al.*, 1990; Spring *et al.*, 1991; Noble *et al.*, submitted; and unpublished data), including two studies with 3 months treatment and one month of post-treatment evaluation and two studies of 6 months duration, one of which (Noble *et al.*, submitted) had a 12-month follow-up period, included well-validated mood rating scales in addition to measures of appetite and weight. There were no differences between dF and placebo-treated patients on mood scales, and there was no evidence of treatment-emergent or post-treatment depression.

Ten studies (Silverstone *et al.*, 1987; Finer *et al.*, 1988; Guy-Grand *et al.*, 1989; Spring *et al.*, 1991; Wurtman *et al.*, 1993; Noble *et al.*, submitted; and unpublished data), using sleep rating scales (e.g. Stanford Sleepiness Scale) including the 12-month INDEX study and the Noble Long-Term study (Noble *et al.*, submitted) (with 6 months treatment and 12 months follow-up), found no significant differences between dF and placebo in sleep quality. Mild day-time sedation was seen occasionally but resolved with continued treatment. No effects on sleep were observed post treatment.

Three studies (Spring *et al.*, 1991; Noble *et al.*, submitted; and unpublished data) included various tests of attention, concentration, mental function, executive function and memory; no significant dF/placebo differences were observed. For example, the Noble Long-Term study, employing the Mini Mental State Examination found no scores outside normal values and no dF/placebo differences either at the end of 6 months of treatment or during 12 months of post-treatment follow-up. These findings are in agreement with published reports where dF or *dl*-F treatments did not induce adverse neuropsychological effects (Ho *et al.*, 1986; Blouin *et al.*, 1988; Baud *et al.*, 1989; Ekman *et al.*, 1989; Oades *et al.*, 1990; Stern *et al.*, 1990; Aman *et al.*, 1993; Fahy *et al.*, 1993; Grunberger *et al.*, 1993; Hetem *et al.*, 1993; Bond *et al.*, 1995).

Three studies (unpublished) using structured neurological assessments found no indication of adverse neurological signs with up to 3 months treatment and 1 month of post-treatment follow-up.

The results of this review indicate that at the clinical dose recommended for the treatment of obesity, dF is safe and well tolerated and is without risk of acute or delayed adverse effects involving the central nervous system. These findings are in concert with clinical experience comprised of over 10 million patient exposures that indicate a benign side effects profile and a favourable risk/benefit ratio for dF.

POST-MARKETING INFORMATION – PHARMACOVIGILANCE DATA

Dexfenfluramine was approved for the treatment of obesity in France in December 1985 and thereafter was approved and launched in 65 other countries. A crude estimate of patient exposure to dF has been calculated from the sales volumes and corresponds to 41 505 000 patient-months until November 1995.

Table 1 presents the main side effects collected in all spontaneous and clinical trial reports, published or unpublished, and received by Servier Pharmacovigilance Department from worldwide sources between December 1985 and November 1995. Spontaneous reports included all individual case reports sent spontaneously to the Medical Departments of Servier by health-care professionals, including those received from Regulatory Authorities and those published in the medical literature. From clinical trials, only those leading to drug discontinuations for medical reasons with a reasonable possibility that the drug may play a role, are reported.

The cases have been classified by body system. The most frequent reported side effects are in agreement with the safety profile derived from clinical trials (fatigue, diarrhoea, nausea, headache, dizziness, sedation). Most of these effects were observed at the beginning of the treatment, were very mild in intensity and disappeared rapidly.

The side effects included in the 'nervous system' section appear to reflect the pharmacological properties of the drug (unlike other anorectic compounds, therapeutic doses of dF do not induce CNS stimulant effects) and present similarities with the side effect profile of selective serotonin reuptake inhibitors (SSRI) (Mitchell, 1994). Most of the reactions appear to be minor, subjective and often transient.

In contrast, severe cases of pulmonary hypertension were reported in patients exposed to dexfenfluramine. Spontaneous reports occurred in Europe (essentially in France and Belgium). However, it has to be noted that cases without evidence of underlying cardiopulmonary or collagen vascular diseases and appropriate timing were rarely observed (reporting rate: 1:718 000 patient-months in France).

A European epidemiological case control study (International Primary Pulmonary Hypertension Study, IPPHS) was conducted between October 1992 and September 1994. The results have been published (Abenhaim *et al.*, 1996) and presented to the European (EMEA) and American (FDA) Health Authorities. The study shows a statistically significant association between Primary Pulmonary Hypertension (PPH) and all anorectic agents (amphetamine derivatives and fenfluramine), when used for more than 3 months (odds ratio of 23.1). A significant association was also shown with obesity itself (BMI > 30).

Table 1

Main adverse effects reported spontaneously between December 1985 and November 1995

Adverse drug reactions (observed on drug or after withdrawal)	Dexfenfluramine worldwide
Body as a whole	
Headache	190
Fatigue/asthenia	127
Malaise	52
Oedema	47
Chills/rigors	23
Cardiovascular system	
Faintness/syncope	35
Systemic hypertension	32
Hypotension	25
Migraine	21
Digestive system	
Diarrhoea	207
Nausea	163
Abdominal colic/pain	68
Dry mouth	55
Vomiting	60
Liver disorders	29
Nervous system	
Dizziness	164
Sedation/somnolence	150
Depression	90
Vertigo	65
Confusion	52
Insomnia	53
Anxiety	41
Paraesthesia	32
Nervousness/excitation	35
Agitation	28
Tremor	24
Diplopia	19
Hallucination/paroniria	28
Ataxia	10
Concentration impairment	26
Coordination abnormal	5
Libido decreased	6
Skin and appendages	
Dermatitis/rash	46
Pruritus	40
Urticaria	39
Alopecia	23
Special senses	
Vision abnormal/blurred	33
Mydriasis	45
Urogenital system	
Impotence	14
Urinary frequency	26

However, it should be remembered that the absolute risk is low (background rate of the disease: 1–2 per million), and that direct relationship between use of anorectic drugs and PPH remains uncertain.

In summary, dexfenfluramine appears to be well tolerated. There is no clinical relevance of the neurochemical changes induced by high doses in some animal studies. Moreover, overall benefit/risk ratio is highly favourable and should be improved by careful respect of the indications, exclusion of the non-responders to treatment, and close surveillance of pulmonary symptoms.

REFERENCES

Abenhaim L, Moride Y, Brenot F *et al*. (1996) Appetite-suppressant drugs and the risk of pulmonary hypertension. *New Eng. J. Med.* **335**: 609–616.

Aman M, Kern R, McGhee D, Arnold L. (1993) Fenfluramine and Methylphenidate in children with mental retardation and attention deficit hyperactivity disorder: Laboratory effects. *J Autism Dev Disor* **23**: 491–506.

Baud P, Le Roch K, Sebban C (1989) Effects EEG quantifiés et psychométriques de 3 doses de dexfenfluramine chez l'adulte jeune. *Neurophysiol Clin* **19**: 241–255.

Blouin A, Blouin J, Perez E *et al*. (1988) Treatment of bulimia with fenfluramine and desipramine. *J Clin Psychopharmacol* **8**: 261–269.

Bond A, Feizollah S, Lader M (1995) The effects of D-fenfluramine on mood and performance, and on neuroendocrine indicators of 5-HT function. *J Psychopharmacol* **9**: 1–8.

Brzezinski AA, Wurtman JJ, Wurtman RJ *et al*. (1990) D-fenfluramine suppresses the increased calorie and carbohydrate intakes and improves the mood of women with premenstrual depression. *Obst Gynecol* **76**: 296–301.

Ekman G, Miranda-Linne F, Gillberg C *et al*. (1989) Fenfluramine treatment of twenty children with autism. *J Autism Dev Disord* **19**: 511–532.

Fahy T, Eisler I, Russell G (1993) A placebo-controlled trial of d-fenfluramine in bulimia nervosa. *Br J Psychiat* **162**: 597–603.

Finer N, Craddock D, Lavielle R, Keen H (1988) Effect of 6 months therapy with dexfenfluramine in obese patients: studies in the United Kingdom. *Clin Neuropharmacol* **11**: S179–S186.

Finer N, Finer S, Naoumova RP (1989) Prolonged use of a very low calorie diet (Cambridge diet) in massively obese patients attending an obesity clinic: Safety, efficacy and additional benefit from dexfenfluramine. *Int J Obesity* **13**: 91–93.

Guy-Grand B, Apfelbaum M, Crepaldi G *et al*. (1989) International trial of long-term dexfenfluramine in obesity. *Lancet* 1142–1145.

Guy-Grand B, Apfelbaum M, Crepaldi G *et al*. (1990) Effect of withdrawal of dexfenfluramine on body weight and food intake after one year's administration. *Int J Obesity* **14**: abstract 1F-4.

Grunberger J, Saletu B, Linzmayer L, Barbanoj M (1993) Clinical-pharmacological study with the two isomers (*d-*, *l-*) of fenfluramine and its comparison with chlorpromazine and *d*-amphetamine: Psychometric and psychophysiological evaluation. *Meth Find Exp Clin Pharmacol* **15**: 313–328.

Hetem L, de-Souza C, Guiramaes F *et al*. (1993) D-fenfluramine reduces anxiety induced by stimulated public speaking. *Brazilian J Med Biol Res* **26**: 971–974.

Ho H, Lockitch G, Eaves L, Jacobson B (1986) Blood serotonin concentrations and fenfluramine therapy in autistic children. *J Pediatr* **108**(3): 465–469.

Mitchell PB (1994) Selective serotonin reuptake inhibitors: Adverse effects, toxicity and interactions. *Adv Drug React Toxicol Rev* **13**: 121–144.

Noble RE, Sabounjian LA, Gammans R (1996) Effects of dexfenfluramine on CNS function in obese patients. (Submitted for publication.)

Oades R, Stern L, Walker M *et al.* (1990) Event-related potentials and monoamines in autistic children on a clinical trial of fenfluramine. *Int J Psychophysiol* **8**: 197–212.

O'Rourke D, Wurtman JJ, Wurtman RJ *et al.* (1989) Treatment of seasonal depression with d-fenfluramine. *J Clin Psychiat* **50**: 343–347.

Silverstone T, Smith G, Richards R (1987) A comparative evaluation of dextrofenfluramine and dl-fenfluramine on hunger, food intake, psychomotor function and side-effects in normal human volunteers. In: Bender AE and Brooks LJ (eds). *Body Weight Control. The Physiology, Clinical Treatment and Prevention of Obesity.* Churchill Livingstone, London: 240–246.

Spring B, Wurtman J, Gleason R *et al.* (1991) Weight gain and withdrawal symptoms after smoking cessation: A preventive intervention using d-fenfluramine. *Health Psychol* **10**: 216–223.

Stern L, Walker M, Sawyer M *et al.* (1990) A controlled crossover trial of fenfluramine in autism. *J Child Psychol Psychiat* **31**: 569–585.

Wurtman J, Wurtman R, Reynolds S *et al.* (1987) Fenfluramine suppresses snack intake among carbohydrate cravers but not among non carbohydrate cravers. *Int J Eating Dis* **6**: 687–699.

Wurtman J, Wurtman R, Berry E *et al.* (1993) Dexfenfluramine, fluoxetine and weight loss among female carbohydrate cravers. *Neuropsychopharmacol* **93**: 201–210.

Part IV

Benefit/Risk Ratio of the Treatment of Obesity

Benefits and Risks of Treating Obesity

Theodore B. VanItallie

Professor Emeritus of Medicine, Columbia University, College of Physicians and Surgeons, New York, NY, USA

When the benefits and risks of treating obesity are being considered, we must first determine whether estimation of a benefit/risk ratio is for the purpose of making a public health policy decision or whether we are attempting to arrive at a judgement about treatment of an individual patient.

At the public policy level, we are beginning to be able to develop increasingly reliable estimates of the excess morbidity and mortality attributable to overweight in the US. Such estimates are derived from the calculation of values for Population Attributable Risk per cent (PAR%), which can be defined as the proportion of disease in a population attributable to the exposure (Hennekens and Buring, 1987). An example of a PAR% would be the proportion of hypertension in a population attributable to obesity. However, it is hazardous to apply a PAR% derived from the experience with one population to another, disparate population.

Using the PAR% of 20 for hypertension proposed by Colditz in 1992, one can estimate that there are currently about 8.6 million US adults whose hypertension is attributable to obesity (20% of 43.2 million US adults with hypertension during 1988–91 (Burt *et al.*, 1995)). It also appears that a high proportion (*c.* 80%) of non-insulin-dependent diabetes mellitus (NIDDM) is attributable to overweight (T.B. VanItallie and J.E. Manson, unpublished research). Using this PAR%, one can estimate that overweight is responsible for 9.4 million cases of NIDDM among US adults (80% of the 11.7 million people believed to suffer from NIDDM (American Diabetes Association, 1993)).

In a 16-year follow-up of 115 195 participants in the Nurses' Health Study (NHS), Manson *et al.* (1995) documented 4726 deaths that had occurred in

T. B. VanItallie

Table 1.
BMI and all-cause mortality risk

BMI Category (kg m^{-2})	Multivariate relative risk	Attributable risk (%)
<19	1.0	0.0
19–<22	1.2	16.7
22–<25	1.2	16.7
25–<27	1.3	23.1
27–<29	1.6	37.5
29–<32	2.1	52.4
≥32	2.2	54.5

Adapted from Manson *et al.* (1995), with permission.

this cohort from the study's inception through 1992. In an analysis of all-cause mortality in a subset limited to weight-stable, never-smoking women excluding the first 4 years of follow-up, Manson *et al.* calculated the relative risk of dying and the attributable risk for seven categories of body mass index (BMI). The findings are given in Table 1.

As the table shows, more than 50% of all-cause deaths occurring in the women with BMIs ≥29 kg m^{-2} were attributable to their overweight. The overall PAR% for the weight-stable, non-smoking NHS participants, after exclusion of the first 4 years of follow-up, was 23.3. In view of the high attributable risk values shown in Table 1, it is noteworthy that about 34.7 million US men and women 20–74 years of age have BMIs ≥30 kg m^{-2} (National Center for Health Statistics, 1995).

If a certain amount of morbidity and mortality can be attributed to overweight/obesity, it follows that, to the extent overweight/obesity can be prevented, the excess morbidity and mortality attributable to this condition will be correspondingly reduced. However, because the damaging effects of obesity on health appear to accumulate over time, the degree to which sustained therapeutic weight reduction can reverse these adverse effects is difficult to predict. Nevertheless, beneficial effects of intentional weight loss on health and longevity have been reported. Thus, among the participants in the NHS, women who lost more than 5.0 kg between the age of 18 and the inception of the study in 1976 (12 to 37 years later) had a substantially reduced risk for NIDDM (Colditz *et al.*, 1995). Intentional weight loss of any amount has also been associated with an appreciable reduction in mortality risk in never-smoking women with obesity-related conditions (Williamson *et al.*, 1995).

Goldstein (1992) has reviewed the literature on the medical effects of modest weight reduction (≤10%) in obese patients with such co-morbidities as

NIDDM, hypertension or hyperlipidaemia. He concludes his review with the following comment: 'A large proportion of obese patients with NIDDM, hypertension, and hyperlipidemia experience positive benefits with modest weight loss.'

Although there are good reasons to believe that therapeutic weight reduction can contribute to the alleviation of such conditions as angina pectoris, congestive heart failure and obstructive sleep apnoea, it is virtually impossible to quantify beneficial effects of this kind. Nevertheless, clinicians have to be aware of potentially favourable effects of weight loss like these on clinical status and they cannot be ignored when risks are being weighed against benefits.

The treatment of obesity is frequently eclectic, with the obese patient being offered a programme that includes a reduced-calorie diet, an exercise regimen and also prescription of an anti-obesity drug. There are certain risks asso-

Table 2

Some modifiers of BMI-associated morbidity and/or mortality risk

Abaters	Augmenters
Lower body (femoral-gluteal) fat distribution pattern	Upper body (abdominal) fat distribution pattern
Ostensibly good health	Impaired health
Absence of obesity-related risk factors and/or co-morbidities	Presence of one or more obesity-related risk factors and/or co-morbidities
Middle-aged or elderly	Young adult (20–45 years of age)
Female	Male
Absence of a family history of obesity-relevant illness	Presence of a family history of obesity-relevant illness
Obesity of brief duration	Obesity of prolonged duration
Membership in a race not known to be vulnerable to obesity-associated health problems	Membership in a race known to be vulnerable to obesity-associated health problems (e.g., NIDDM vulnerability in obese Pima Indians).
Above normal stature	Below normal stature

Adapted from VanItallie and Lew (1992), with permission.

ciated with weight loss *per se*, particularly if the rate of weight loss is too
rapid. In rare instances, rapid, massive weight loss can give rise to potentially
lethal ventricular arrhythmias. Anti-obesity drugs can also have serious side
effects; for example, it has been estimated that any use of anorectics is
associated with an increased risk (odds ratio for any exposure 6.3) of developing primary pulmonary hypertension (PPH), a very rare but extremely serious
disorder that, in the general population, occurs at a rate of about 1–2 cases per
million persons per year (L. Abenhaim *et al.*, 1996).

As Table 1 indicates, the risk of dying attributable to obesity rises rapidly in
NHS women with BMIs ≥27. At a BMI ≥29, attributable risk per cent
(AR%) already exceeds 50. Hence, the obese patients most likely to be treated
with anorectics are also those who are already at high risk of dying from an
obesity-attributable illness. In such cases, the benefit/risk ratio is clearly
favourable, assuming that anorectic treatment is effective in promoting weight
reduction and preventing weight regain. Of course, such benefit/risk esti-
mations will remain problematic until long-term cohort studies can demonstrate that the risk of dying from an obesity-attributable cause diminishes
systematically as body weight is decreased, and then remains stable during
maintenance of the reduced weight.

When it comes to making an assessment of the benefits and risks of treating
an individual obese patient, the physician should consider various risk-
modifying factors such as those shown in Table 2.

It is not enough to make a judgement based solely on the 'average'
attributable risk associated with a particular BMI. A patient's morbidity and/
or mortality risk (and hence the urgency of treatment) is likely to be increased
by the presence of one or more of the augmenters shown in the table.
Conversely, if abaters predominate, the patient's risk is likely to be correspondingly reduced.

REFERENCES

Abenhaim L, Moride Y, Brenot F *et al*. (1996) Appetite suppressant drugs and the risk
   of primary pulmonary hypertension. *New Engl. J. Med.* **335**: 609–616.
American Diabetes Association (1993) *Diabetes 1993 Vital Statistics*
Burt VL, Whelton P, Roculla EJ *et al*. (1995) Prevalence of hypertension in the U.S.
   adult population. Results from the third National Health and Nutrition Examin-
   ation Survey, 1988–1991. *Hypertension* **25**: 205–213.
Colditz GA (1992) Economic costs of obesity. *Am J Clin Nutr* **55**: 503S-507S
Colditz GA, Willett WC, Rotmisky A, Manson JE (1995) Weight gain as a risk factor
   for clinical diabetes in women. *Ann Intern Med* **122**: 481–486.
Goldstein DF (1992) Beneficial health effects of modest weight loss. *Int J Obesity* **16**:
   397–415.
Hennekens CH, Buring JE (1987) *Epidemiology in Medicine*. Little Brown,
   Boston.

Manson JE, Willett, WC, Stampfer MJ *et al.* (1995) Body weight and mortality in women. *New Engl J Med* **333**: 677–685.

National Center for Health Statistics (1995) *Health, United States, 1994.* Public Health Service, Hyattsville, Maryland.

VanItallie TB, Lew EA (1992). Assessment of morbidity and mortality risk in the overweight patient. In: Wadden TA and VanItallie TB (eds) *Treatment of the Seriously Obese Patient.* Guilford, New York: 3–32.

Williamson DF, Pamuk E, Thun M *et al.* (1995) Prospective study of intentional weight loss and mortality in never-smoking US white women aged 40–64 years. *Am J Epidemiol* **114**: 1128–1141.

Round Table Discussion

T. B. VanItallie, M. Apfelbaum, R. L. Atkinson,
C. Bouchard, G. A. Bray, G. A. Faich, B. Guy-Grand,
A. J. Stunkard and S. Nicolaïdis

T. B. VanItallie: I have prepared some questions for each member of the panel. After they have been addressed we shall open the discussion to the floor and let everyone participate.

As a starting point, I would like to call on Dr. Bray for any comments he wants to make on the issue of obesity hazards.

G. A. Bray: In his remarks, Mr. Essner appropriately outlined the co-morbid major risk factors including the cardiovascular effects, the diabetic effects, and the dyslipidaemias.

T. B. VanItallie: Yes, but obesity also aggravates a host of medical problems such as angina, congestive heart failure, respiratory insufficiency, and musculo-skeletal disorders. All this adds up to an enormous health burden attributable to obesity.

I'll go on now to Dr. Bouchard; and ask him to comment on peculiarities that modulate the risk of obesity. We've been talking about body mass indices as independent variables, but we cannot just limit our evaluation to a person's body mass index.

C. Bouchard: Thanks Ted. There are certainly factors that can aggravate a patient's adverse response to obesity – the saturated fat content of the diet would be one example. But I would like to emphasize particularly the fat distribution issue because this is one on which we are beginning to acquire revealing data. When we look at the relationship between total body fat, and markers of morbid conditions, we see that, versus total body fat, there is always a slightly higher correlation between the amount of abdominal visceral fat, and, for example, markers of insulin resistance or dislipidaemia. This doesn't mean that visceral fat is the main culprit, but only that this small fat depot is located strategically near the liver where it exerts a greater influence than any other fat depot in the human body. The discouraging news is that the correlation between visceral fat and total body fat is only moderate. So normal-weight people may have a fairly high level of visceral fat; and the converse. The good news is that when you lose weight you tend to lose visceral fat. It appears to be one of the more readily mobilized fat depots. And the last bit of good news is that visceral fat is mobilized substantially by dexfenfluramine. There aren't very many studies on this but we do have a good one from Sharon Marx *et al.* from Australia. Their experiment shows that with a very small amount of weight loss, only three kilograms over twelve weeks, the subjects lost 33% of their visceral fat content as measured by MRI. The same subjects lost only 10% of their subcutaneous fat depot. This study indicates that weight loss combined with drug intervention can alter the co-morbidity situation quite significantly.

T. B. VanItallie: Thank you Claude. Dr. Atkinson has done some important studies on the long-term treatment of obesity and the problem of preventing recidivism. Dick, would you speak about the health benefits of long-term treatment?

R. L. Atkinson: Several of the speakers have commented on the improvements in blood pressure, blood sugar, haemoglobin A1C, and blood lipid levels that accompany weight loss, but there are not a lot of data to show that they can be sustained. However, Guy-Grand showed continuity with blood pressure, cholesterol, and triglycerides after one year of treatment with dexfenflura-mine. Weintraub's data, over two years, revealed that lipid levels were improved on obesity treatment and that the improvement was sustained as long as weight loss persisted. The data show that when people come off obesity drugs, they regain their weight. The drugs may not cause a large weight loss, but they certainly cause some weight loss. Even modest weight loss appears to cause long-term improvement in some of the co-morbid conditions. In our hands, two years of treatment with phentermine and dexfenfluramine confirm these sustained improvements. Dr. Guy-Grand has shown the same thing in the INDEX study using only dexfenfluramine. Therefore, I think the chances of keeping down the co-morbid conditions are better with obesity drugs than with just diet, exercise, and behaviour modification.

T. B. VanItallie: Thank you very much Dick. Dr. Stunkard was one of the first people, if not the first, to show conclusively the importance of heredity in the determination of the body mass index, using twin studies. He is probably as impressed as anybody with the importance of family history as a risk factor for the development of obesity. I'd like to ask him whether he has any thoughts on how we can detect people who are particularly at risk of becoming obese, and whether there are any new approaches to this detection process.

A. J. Stunkard: Our data suggest that dexfenfluramine can reduce the binge eating disorder. In light of this data, bulimia nervosa may also be reduced which may indicate substantial use of the drug by psychiatrists. We certainly need more developmental studies to make sure. As Claude Bouchard said, we have a pretty good idea from family history who is at high risk. And it's particularly people with two obese parents. If we assume that approximately one-third of Americans are fat and if they don't exhibit assortive mating, then only one-ninth of the population would be at risk, which is a more manageable number. The NHANES finding of an increase in obesity in children suggests another target population, namely, people who are already obese. There's a huge increase in the prevalence of obesity among children in the United States. This increase is not evenly distributed across the spectrum, but concentrated among people who are already obese. So there are two ways of identifying target populations, one from parental obesity, and then from your own obesity. This particular method was used in a study by Laura Lissner reported a few months ago that impressed me enormously. She looked at the weight gain over a period of time of four groups of people as a function of increasing fat in the diet. Her four groups were thin people with thin parents, fat people with thin parents, thin people with fat parents, and fat people with fat parents. She saw that as the fat content of the diet increased moderately, there was really no change in the increase in bodyweight until you got to 4.9 MJ day^{-1} of fat. At that point, the group of people who were obese with obese parents had a very powerful threshold effect but the other three groups didn't show much effect. There was a weight gain over approximately five years of eight body mass units, or 20+ kg. This study suggests a way of not only identifying a target population, but also a target behaviour. So I think this is a very exciting prospect for the future.

T. B. VanItallie: Thank you Mickey. There are at least two ways of looking at benefit–risk ratios. One is the kind of decision that has to be made at the public policy level. For example, the Food and Drug Administration made such a judgement when they approved the marketing of Dexfenfluramine, knowing both the risks and the benefits. The second kind of decision is the more personal or individual judgement, made by a physician when he/she sees a patient and must determine how serious the problem of obesity is for that patient and what kinds of treatment are appropriate. Dr. Apfelbaum has been prominent in giving advice to government agencies about risks and benefits; I would like to ask Marian if he would comment about the processes of reasoning by which one arrives at a benefit–risk decision.

M. Apfelbaum: Thank you. About twenty years ago there was a decision, in France, that since all anorectic drugs were supposed to be addictive, none should be used for more than three weeks. The nonaddictive character of dexfenfluramine brought about a specific regulation according to which this drug could be prescribed for a period of three months instead of three weeks. Dexfenfluramine was so successful that a lot of people, obese and not so obese, were taking the drug. Three years ago Deroux reported that in a series of fifty people with primary pulmonary hypertension (PPH), more than twelve were users of anorectic drugs, including dexfenfluramine. This provoked a substantial change in the official mood. Servier did a very good job in helping to organize a massive study of this problem. The conclusion of this study is that the use of any anorectic drug, including dexfenfluramine, results in a relative risk of developing PPH of 6.3. PPH is a very rare disease with one or two cases arising per million individuals. However, I have proposed that an anorectic drug should not be used if the subject has a body mass index of less than thirty. Secondly, the first prescription must be issued by a physician within a public hospital, and without payment to the prescribing specialist. Once the patient has the prescription, s/he returns to the care of the general practitioner. After three months the practitioner must decide if the drug is working. If s/he thinks it is, s/he now has the responsibility of following the patient's treatment. The previous three-month law has now been abolished, and treatment is often continued for many years. However, this law was abolished only for dexfenfluramine, and not for other anorectic drugs. This is because risk of addiction to dexfenfluramine is not a concern.

T. B. VanItallie: Thank you Marian. Next I'd like to ask Gerry Faich where he thinks we should be going now with the benefit–risk issue as it applies to dexfenfluramine. We are certainly going to be facing discussions of this sort when the inevitable cases of anorexigen-triggered primary pulmonary hypertension emerge. Enunciation of a sound approach to this complex issue would help us all to develop a better understanding of how one arrives at a defensible benefit–risk judgement. Would you like to comment on that Gerry?

G. A. Faich: I would say that it is perfectly clear that we're dealing with a situation where the risk is perceived of as an added risk. That is, it's an error of commission. The benefits of the drug have to be seen as preventative. Firstly, we need to understand that we're dealing with risk definition; how big is the risk? How much do we know about it? What is our ongoing continual monitoring? Because of course the whole issue has been historically that dexfenfluramine is not aminorex. We are not sitting on the cusp of an incipient epidemic, and that is absolutely a critical and continuing issue. There isn't going to be a need to continually collect cases and deal with them. The second issue, and somewhat embedded in the first, is how do you communicate a risk? How do you talk about a very rare risk in a meaningful way to both clinicians and patients? Risk avoidance and risk perception are not linear kinds of relationships at all. It behooves the sponsors, as well as clinicians, to do what they can to put this risk in perspective. Once you understand that obesity is not only a chronic and resistant disease, but is very directly associated with mortality consequences, your perception of the disease itself begins to change and the parameters that go with perceiving what is an acceptable risk. Those are critical issues that are going to continue to be part of the launch and subsequent use of the drug for some years to come. The issue will not go away. From a clinician's viewpoint we need to understand that every drug has its risks, and its benefits. We want to select for treatment a population in which the benefits will be maximized and risks minimized. The labelling on the drug indicates quite clearly that it needs to be reserved for people who have failed on a diet and who have reached a level of obesity where predictably, they will sustain the considerable risks and hazards of obesity itself. Also, when a 'non-responder' is identified, the drug should be stopped because there is potentially no benefit, and you can't justify the risk.

T. B. VanItallie: Thank you Gerry. There is still progress to be made to teach not only lay people but physicians about the hazards of obesity.

T. B. VanItallie: I'm going to now call on the president, Dr. Nicolaidis, to close the meeting, and make his final comments.

S. Nicolaidis: Thank you Ted. At this late hour I will take a minute or two to remind you that, just as Silvio Garattini said, we feel like a scientific family working on long-term treatment of obesity and assessing the various actions of dexfenfluramine. It's amazing how prominent investigators like all of you – physicians and scientists – manage to continue to report impressive new data. Taken in aggregate, your findings continue to demonstrate that dexfenfluramine is one of the most versatile and complex molecules that I for one have ever encountered. It's incredible how many targets this molecule can reach during a treatment. Because it's so effective, dexfenfluramine has attracted much interest, also many advocates and, inevitably, some enemies. It is not just by chance that this molecule has become such an important drug as well as an instrument of investigation. Servier, and now Interneuron and Wyeth-Ayerst, are companies that understood pharmacological research not only leads to the discovery of therapeutically useful molecules, but also that through the study of the action of such molecules – in this case dexfenfluramine – we have been able to enhance our understanding of the physiology of hunger and satiety, of energy metabolism, and of the role and behaviour of the adipose tissue and its stored triglycerides. The laboratory and clinical investigations sponsored and encouraged by Servier have laid the foundation for the work reported here today and have made possible the recent approval of dexfenfluramine by the U.S. Food and Drug Administration. We are thankful for this philosophy of Servier (and now Interneuron and Wyeth-Ayerst) which has generated so much research, and a more scientific approach to a remarkable therapeutic molecule.

Printed and bound by CPI Group (UK) Ltd, Croydon, CR0 4YY

08/10/2024

01042201-0001